HOW
HOCKEY
CAN SAVE
HEALTHCARE

A Principle-Based Approach to Reforming the
Canadian Healthcare System

Stephen Pinney MD

Lulu Publishing Services rev. date: 7/26/2016

To Canadian patients: past, present, and future

CONTENTS

LIST OF ABBREVIATIONS

AAMC	Association of American Medical Colleges
ABF	Activity-Based Funding
ABJHI	Alberta Bone and Joint Health Institute
ALC	Alternative Level of Care
AO	Arbeitsgemeinschaft für Osteosynthesefragen (Association for the Study of Internal Fixation)
AUC	appropriate use criteria
BC	British Columbia
BNA	British North America Act
CBC	Canadian Broadcasting Corporation
CCF	Cooperative Commonwealth Federation
CHA	Canadian Hockey Association
CHSRF	Centre for Health Services Research Foundation
CHT	Canada Health Transfer
CIHI	Canadian Institute for Health Information
CMA	Canadian Medical Association
CPG	clinical practice guidelines
CQI	continuous quality improvement
CT	computed tomography scan
DRG	Diagnostic Related Group
EKG	electrocardiogram
EMR	Electronic Medical Record
ENT	Ear, Nose, and Throat
EOC	episode of care
FAA	Federal Aviation Administration

FMEA	failure modes and effects analysis
GDP	gross domestic product
GPs	General Practitioners
HIDS	Hospital Insurance and Diagnostic Services Act
HIV	human immunodeficiency virus
ICER	incremental cost-effectiveness ratio
ICU	intensive care unit
IHI	Institute for Healthcare Improvement
IHL	International Hockey League
IOM	Institute of Medicine
IPU	Integrated Practice Unit
IT	information technology
LPN	Licensed Practical Nurse
LTC	long-term care
MA	Medical Assistant
MSC	Medical Services Commission
MSK	musculoskeletal
MRI	Magnetic Resonance Imaging
NCEPOD	London: National Confidential Enquiry into Perioperative Deaths
NHA	National Hockey Association
NHL	National Hockey League
NHS	National Health Service (British)
NP	Nurse Practitioner
NSQIP	North American Surgical Quality Improvement Program
OECD	Organization for Economic Co-operation and Development
OPD	outpatient department
OPHL	Ontario Professional Hockey League
OR	operating room
PA	Physician's Assistant
PCHA	Pacific Coast Hockey Association
PCMH	patient-centred medical home

PDCA	Plan-Do-Check-Act cycle
PFCC	patient and family centred care methodology
QI	Quality Improvement
RCA	Root Cause Analysis
RN	Registered Nurse
SCAMP	standardized clinical assessment and management plan
SQC	Statistical Quality Control
SSC	Specialists Services Committee
STIs	sexually transmitted infections
TNSE	True North Sports and Entertainment
TQM	Total Quality Management
USSR	Union of Soviet Socialist Republics (Soviet Union)
UTI	urinary tract infections
VA	Veterans Affairs (Veteran's Health Administration)
WOW II	Who Operates When

INTRODUCTION

I had an office, but no fax or printer.

It's funny how small things can have big impacts. There I was, on the first day of my new job as the head of the orthopaedic department at a large Canadian hospital, and I was stumped by a printer. Or lack thereof.

"No problem!" I thought. I will simply walk down the street to the office supply store and purchase one. "I am sorry, but you can't do that!" my new assistant informed me. Apparently all hospital equipment, including faxes and printers, had to be purchased, installed, and maintained by the hospital's information technology (IT) team. They placed an expedited order, and the waiting began.

I phoned the IT department daily for the first week. Each time, I spoke with a different person, each of whom was friendly but unable to help me. I phoned three times in the second week. By the fourth week, I gave up calling altogether. Sometime during the fifth week, two men arrived unannounced, installed my printer, and left. I finally had a printer.

What does obtaining a printer have to do with providing high-quality, cost-effective health care? Nothing and everything! Nothing, because as a physician, I do not need a printer to assess, diagnose, and treat a patient. Everything, because good modern medical care is predicated on successfully integrating the entire series of events that comprise each patient's episode of care (EOC). For example, the typical surgical EOC consists of all events from the decision to proceed with surgery until the patient's recovery from that surgery—often months after the procedure itself. Each event within the patient's EOC is interrelated, and problems with one segment of the EOC can (and often do) affect the patient's outcome and/or the cost of providing care. A fax machine allowed me to receive referrals, x-ray reports, laboratory results, and a variety of other communications necessary for me to effectively do my job as a surgeon. The world of healthcare remains archaic in many ways, and as such, a fax may be the only way I will know that a patient on whom I operated has shown up at an outside emergency room with a problem. A functioning printer and fax machine are therefore two of the many essential elements needed to ensure a successful EOC.

If only this type of siloed, dysfunctional organization had been confined to the IT department, things might have been OK, but it was everywhere. Inefficiency and structural roadblocks were built into the fabric and culture of the Canadian healthcare system. The system has been designed, albeit unintentionally, to fail. What I witnessed during my two years working in the Canadian healthcare system stunned me and compelled me to write this book. It is written for those who are interested in an improved understanding of the existing system and what we as Canadians can do to realize the true potential of the system. And it is written for taxpayers and patients who deserve better.

My premise in writing this book is that the Canadian healthcare system is prohibitively expensive yet struggles to deliver even mediocre care—not because bad people are running the system, but because of the system itself. All systems are perfectly organized to achieve the results they get, and the Canadian healthcare system is no different.[1] The "system" is a prisoner to its history. It coalesced almost fifty years ago as a means of funding a way of practicing medicine that no longer applies in today's modern medical world.

I grew up in Kingston, Ontario, and did my medical school training at McGill University in Montreal. In 1991, I headed west to the University of British Columbia, where I completed my orthopaedic residency training. However, like many of my resident colleagues training during the 1990s (and today), the Canadian job market for orthopaedic surgeons was barren, and a move to the United States offered greater opportunities. After honing my clinical and surgical skills for a decade, I began to look for a greater challenge.

---

[1]   This idea has been attributable to various authors including David Hanna, Paul Plsek, and even Albert Einstein. Within the healthcare setting the idea has been attributed to Dr. Paul Batalden.

In 2009, after ten years of working as an academic orthopaedic surgeon in the United States, I was recruited to return to Canada. I accepted a leadership position as head of the orthopaedic department at one of the largest hospitals in British Columbia and started work in August of 2010. In addition to my administrative responsibilities, I also ran a full clinical practice in orthopaedics—seeing patients in clinic, performing surgeries, and taking emergency calls. I began my Canadian healthcare adventure with genuine excitement at the prospect of helping to harness two of the real strengths of the Canadian healthcare system: first, all patients have health insurance; second, central oversight of the healthcare system allows for the development of large-scale, efficiently coordinated care projects—at least in theory. Many Canadians take these elements of the Canadian healthcare system for granted. Having worked in other systems, I did not.

The job I was recruited into seemed like it would be a great fit. I'd have numerous opportunities: return to Canada to help provide administrative leadership to an orthopaedic department, coordinate care for patients with musculoskeletal problems in my subspecialty (foot and ankle), and continue to pursue my academic interests (teaching and research). Like the vast majority of Canadians, I embrace the ideals of a well-run, publicly-funded healthcare system providing high-quality, universal healthcare coverage to all Canadians. However, after I arrived, it took less than six months for me to realize what I had walked into—ideals and reality are often two very different things. It took another twelve months to realize that a meaningful system change was not going to materialize from within the existing system. As one of my colleagues told me, "After eighteen months, you will understand the system, and then you just need to determine if you can tolerate it for the rest of your career."

The doctors, nurses, and administrators I worked with were some of the nicest and most committed people I have met. However, they were trapped in a dysfunctional system and powerless to do anything about it. For me it was untenable. I could not face my patients—or myself— knowing I was not only part of the system, but purportedly someone who was helping to lead it. The experience has compelled me to push for meaningful healthcare reform in Canada. I hope the messages contained in this book will stimulate ideas, debate, and ultimately actions that will help usher in fundamental system reform.

To contextualize my discussions regarding the Canadian healthcare system, it is important that the reader understand my philosophy of healthcare provision. *I believe that the primary goal of a healthcare system should be to provide high-value healthcare—care that is patient-centered, high quality, and cost-effective.* Anyone looking at the Canadian healthcare system through a different lens may come to a different conclusion.

This book is divided into nine chapters. The first three chapters explore the existing Canadian healthcare system. Chapter 1 looks at the good…and the not so good, providing an overview of what is working, and what is not. Chapter 2 examines the finances of the healthcare system and argues that healthcare in Canada is not "free", but rather prohibitively expensive. Chapter 3 addresses the quality of care the system delivers; despite the aforementioned strengths of the system, increasing evidence is showing that the system is struggling to even reach mediocrity.

Chapter 4 gives a history of medical care outlining the fundamental changes in the approach to how care is delivered that have occurred during the past two centuries –and in particular during the last two decades. Chapter 5 explores the history of healthcare delivery within the Canadian healthcare system. It is not possible to understand the present system without understanding the past and this chapter reviews how the structural organization of the present-day system was established a half-century ago during a time when the practice of medicine was very different than it is today.

Chapter 6 reviews the principles that serve as the foundation of a modern healthcare system. These accepted principles of modern healthcare delivery have been well delineated by healthcare scholars and have been battle-tested in different healthcare systems and other service industries, such as airlines and hotel chains. Chapter 7 outlines how a modern healthcare system needs to be structured—a single governing body; an emphasis on team-based, primary care delivery; coordinated teams to deliver high-value EOCs for more complex problems; and efficiently run healthcare facilities, such as hospitals, where care is actually delivered. In Chapter 8, the principles outlined in Chapter

6 are expanded and applied to the various activities and stakeholders within a healthcare system—the governing bodies (the Ministries of Health, Regional Health authorities, etc.), various healthcare teams, and individual actors within the system (physicians, administrators, etc.).

Chapter 9 presents potential strategies for reforming the Canadian healthcare system. I will argue that the key to reforming the Canadian healthcare system is to reorient the system to ensure it is fully aligned with the accepted principles of modern healthcare delivery that are outlined in Chapter 8. One potential means of achieving fundamental reform is outlined—disruptive innovation in the form of a second parallel public system—a "system within a system" designed from the ground up, based on modern healthcare principles

Fundamental and meaningful healthcare reform will not be an easy task. The reality is that on many levels, the Canadian healthcare system works well for those working within the existing system; many doctors, nurses, healthcare workers, and administrators have carved out well-compensated niches that they protect ferociously. It also works for many Canadians with an idealized view of their healthcare system but no meaningful interaction with the system itself. However, increasing evidence reveals a system that is not working for those on the outside—taxpayers and patients. This final section of the book will explore strategies for reform that truly put the patients and the taxpayers first.

Most chapters have a similar structure. They begin with a hockey scenario—either real or imagined. Comparing the Canadian healthcare system to hockey may seem odd, but it is intended to serve two purposes. First, it provides an analogy to help the reader understand the often opaque workings of what is actually happening within the Canadian healthcare system. Second, the principles and commitments required to successfully run a professional hockey team are similar to those required to run a successful healthcare system. The National Hockey League (NHL) head office is akin to the governing body of a healthcare system. It looks out for the best interests of the league as a whole, and its goals trump those of individual teams. Teams attempt to win games and maintain success throughout the season and into the playoffs.

A successful professional hockey team demonstrates many of the attributes that one would expect to see in a high functioning healthcare team. Both teams set clear goals and select and utilize players to achieve the best outcomes, closely measure their results, and make changes—including personnel changes based on their overall performances. Individual hockey players realize they must be highly skilled and committed to excellence to play hockey professionally. Their individual goals must be subservient to the goals of the team. Similarly, in healthcare, individual practitioners need to work as part of a team so the patient-centered goals of the team trump the personal agendas of doctors and other practitioners. Unfortunately, this is not how the vast majority of the Canadian healthcare system is organized.

There are some important differences in the analogy between hockey and healthcare. One of the most striking is that when a hockey organization functions poorly, their team fails to make the playoffs or is eliminated from the playoffs early, leaving their city and their fans saddened for a day or even a week. When a healthcare system performs poorly, patients suffer—often permanently.

Throughout each chapter, I present stories from the Canadian healthcare system. This represents the view from the healthcare playing field—the ground-level perspective. I experienced these stories firsthand, or in rare instances, had direct knowledge of the events. The names of patients, physicians, and administrators have been changed, and the circumstances altered to protect confidentiality. However, the essential elements of each story are true. An analysis of every story is performed to identify issues or principles.

After reviewing real-life scenarios, background information and facts pertaining to the system as a whole are presented. These discussions aim to provide a broader perspective—the bird's-eye view. Each chapter ends with a return to the hockey analogy, including lessons or ideas we can learn from each analogy that can be applied to the Canadian healthcare system.

Was my experience within the Canadian healthcare system typical? Perhaps the system is working perfectly elsewhere, and I simply witnessed dysfunction in an isolated area. Certainly there is a spectrum of organizations within the Canadian healthcare system. I have no doubt that there are pockets within the system where excellent care is delivered regularly and at a reasonable cost. I have highlighted a number of these examples throughout the book. However, I do believe my experience was representative of the norm. I worked at a hospital that had an excellent reputation and had done well on its accreditation reviews. Yet it was beholden to the same forces that dominate the entire Canadian healthcare system: the same general funding paradigm, the same organizational structure, and the same emphasis (or lack thereof) on the outcomes of care. The problem was the system, and the system was ubiquitous.

When people talk of reforming the Canadian healthcare system, the conversation often moves quickly to opening up a private system, bringing in an "American-style" healthcare system, or changing the source of healthcare funding. These debates are not what this book is about. This book is about how Canadians can make their publicly-funded healthcare system run better—much better!

This book is not intended to push a private Canadian healthcare system, nor is it about importing "American-style" healthcare. It is true that I now practice in the United States and have learned much from their perspectives. However, there is not one style of healthcare delivery in the United States; rather, there are many, very different approaches.[2] The notion that we can describe "American healthcare" as one system is ludicrous. Nevertheless, Canadians can and should look to other health systems, including those in the United States, for aspects of care delivery that work.

How Canadians fund their healthcare system has been open to debate at times. Presently, there is a pseudo-insurance system, with the provincial governments acting as de facto insurance agents. They take in money from taxpayers and disperse this money to those running the health system: administrators and healthcare providers. Unlike insurance companies, they do not demand that users pay a deductible—a

---

[2] Approaches to healthcare delivery in the United States include variations of the traditional fee-for-service approach, a variety of health maintenance organizations (ex. Kaiser and Intermountain Healthcare), a comprehensive workers' compensation system, the Veterans Affairs (VA) hospital system that cares for military personnel and veterans of the military, and an extensive county-based hospital system to help provide for the uninsured and underinsured.

token fee prior to seeing a doctor, receiving surgery, or being admitted to hospital. Such a fee is designed to discourage excessive use of the insurance system, although in some instances it may serve to discourage low-income patients from seeking medical care in a timely manner.

There are definitely right-wing and left-wing views on whether the Canadian system should introduce these types of user fees. Like the private-public debate, such discussions are healthy for the country, regardless of the final decision. However, there is not a right-wing or left-wing way to practice good medical care; politics and national borders do not define the principles of good healthcare delivery. This book does not have a political orientation. It is about how the existing, public Canadian healthcare system can invoke accepted principles of 21st century medical care to dramatically improve the value and quality of the care provided.

It is my hope that this book will stimulate discussion about the problems endemic in the present Canadian healthcare system, and provide a general roadmap for instituting fundamental reform. I encourage the reader to analyze and debate the ideas presented. As Canadians, hockey and healthcare are two of our most prized national treasures. We need to be as passionate about demanding excellence and transparency in Canadian healthcare as we are for demanding quality and success of our favourite professional hockey team. As Canadians, with ingenuity, meaningful reform, hard work, and a focus on the team, we can win the healthcare game.

CHAPTER 1

Overview of the Canadian Healthcare System: The Good... and the Not So Good!

Members of your favourite National Hockey League (NHL) team's organization were interviewed. How do you like the team's prospects?

Reporter: What is your strategy for overseeing this organization?

Owner: Our organization hires good people, nice people, and we have them work within the same system that we have always had. We ensure that they are well-funded. We give them a large block of money at the start of the year—usually 3% or more than they received the year before. The team's results are reviewed regularly, but I am not sure how accurate they are. We rarely fire anyone because we know everyone is trying their best.

Reporter: What is your approach to managing your hockey team?

General Manager: We have a traditional way of doing things here. We have a large management team, and we go to lots of meetings. I don't actually watch any of the hockey games or practices. In fact, the management team and I rarely ever go to the arena. However, we look at lots of reports and lots of data on our computers. Some have questioned the validity of the data, but it looks fine to me.

Reporter: May I speak with your head coach?

General Manager: *Actually, we do not have a head coach. We prefer to have a wide variety of assistant coaches. There is a goalie coach, a left defenseman coach, and a right defenseman coach—even a coach for the hot dog sellers. We try to get these coaches to work together, but they each have their own ideas about how they should do their job. And we accept these differences.*

Reporter: *How did you feel about tonight's hockey game?*

Player: *Great! I was happy with my game tonight.*

Reporter: *But your team lost 6–0.*

Player: *Really, we lost? That's no good! They never tell me the final results. My job is to take face-offs in the second period, and I took a lot of face-offs in the second period tonight. I even managed to win a number of them!*

The Good: Concentrated Clinical Excellence and Universal Coverage

Bone Tumour Conference

For three months in 1992, I was a junior orthopaedic resident assigned to the bone tumour service. Every Monday morning for two hours, I sat in a dimly lit conference room with 6-8 other physicians. It was the British Columbia musculoskeletal tumour conference—an example of concentrated expertise working together as a team. Malignant sarcomas of bone and soft tissues are rare but potentially deadly cancers. This type of tumour claimed the life of Canadian icon Terry Fox.

On one particular Monday, our conference reviewed five patients. Each had been diagnosed with a musculoskeletal tumor during the preceding weeks. These patients, and those who had been reviewed previously, represented every adult patient in the province of British Columbia who had been diagnosed with a malignant musculoskeletal tumour. The health system via the British Columbia Cancer Agency had funneled these patients—or at least their charts, lab results, imaging studies, and pathology reports—into this room where we systematically reviewed them, one by one.

The musculoskeletal oncologist, a physician subspecializing in bone tumours, described the first patient. She specialized in the latest treatment for sarcomas and worked closely with the network of oncologists centered at the various BC Cancer agency sites throughout the province. The patient was a 22-year-old from Kelowna with a three-month history of aching in his knee. X-rays had identified what looked like an aggressive tumour of the distal femur—the thighbone near the knee. A subsequent biopsy was positive for an osteosarcoma—a high-grade tumour of bone. The oncologist described the patient's history and what was found upon physical examination, reviewed the lab results, and outlined the biopsy results. She provided a detailed analysis of the findings that was followed by a discussion among all the team members.

A radiologist specializing in interpreting musculoskeletal images and subspecializing in interpreting x-rays, CT scans, MRI, and bone scans of musculoskeletal tumours gave his opinion. How extensive was the tumour? Did it involve major nerves or vascular structures? Had it metastasized? His approach was calm and systematic, but he spoke with the authority that comes from having reviewed thousands of patient images and that is augmented by a mastery of the latest radiology research. After the radiologist report, the surgeon or oncologist would often ask a pointed question: Does it looks like we can get a clean resection margin and still preserve the sciatic nerve?

The pathologist spoke next, offering a concise review of the pathological analysis of the biopsy: What was the tumour type? Was it high-grade? Did it have any unusual elements? Many general pathologists would see less than five sarcomas a year. The pathologist at the sarcoma conference was seeing five a week; studying them was a central part of his research agenda. He was one of a handful of pathologists in North America with this type of experience and expertise. After his review of the pathology, he fielded questions from the team.

After a robust discussion, the oncologist suggested a treatment course. Further discussions ensued, with everyone making suggestions or challenging assumptions. Ultimately the group all agreed the patient should receive neo-adjuvant chemotherapy—chemotherapy to shrink the tumour prior to attempting a surgical resection. This would be followed by restaging of the tumour—repeating the review that had just occurred, and if a good response had been achieved, then proceeding with surgery to resect the tumour and salvage the limb with a customized knee joint replacement. This is where the orthopaedic service would come in. The attending surgeon I was working with would be asked to perform a complex operation to remove the entire tumour and replace it with a custom knee joint. Very few surgeons performed this uncommon and challenging operation, but for him it was routine.

The above story is an example of one of the truly great things about the Canadian healthcare system—the potential for concentrated excellence working as a team. There is a lot of good in the Canadian healthcare system. Everyone has insurance, so all citizens are eligible for care. Furthermore, everyone has the same insurance, so sending patients between physicians or hospitals is not a problem. Physicians and other healthcare providers are well-trained and generally well-intentioned.

There is also the potential to concentrate expertise, as illustrated by the sarcoma conference.

Canada could—and given how much money is spent, probably *should*—have one of the best healthcare systems in the world. However, Canada doesn't, and according to multiple independent reviews and assessments, it is not even close.[3] The existing system is broken, and the patients and taxpayers of this country are the ones who suffer. What has happened to the Canadian healthcare system? Why has it happened? This book will explore these questions and attempt to determine what Canada can do to reclaim a universal, publicly-funded healthcare system that Canadians can be proud of.

The Not So Good: Financial and Organizational Inefficiency

The Surgical Outpatient Clinic

On any weekday, take a walk through the surgical outpatient clinic at my hospital. Begin walking along the hallway that leads to the clinic, and you will note a line of patients waiting to check in. When they reach the front of the line, they sit down in front of one of the four friendly registration clerks, who proceeds to log their demographic information into a computer registering them for their visit. Walking further, you will see a large group of patients and their families sitting in a waiting room. On a regular basis, a registered nurse will enter the room, call out a name, and escort that patient to an exam room. On the left, you will see another group of patients waiting for their number to be called so they can have an x-ray taken. Turning down another corridor, you will see a series of three- and four-room pods, each containing a doctor who is busy seeing patients.

To the uninitiated, and many administrators, the surgical outpatient department often looks like a busy clinic—the Canadian health system

---

[3]   2014 Commonwealth Report, OECD, etc. list which will be reviewed in Chapter 3.

in action. A closer look reveals a very different story—a story of financial waste, organizational inefficiency, and misdirected or absent goals.

When I take the same walk, I see at least half of the clinic's multimillion-dollar budget wasted. The four friendly registration clerks are collecting patient demographic information that the office staff of each physician has already collected. Rather than institute what would be a normal data transfer in any other industry, the information is collected again when the patient registers.

The registered nurse who takes the patient from the waiting room is being paid close to $100,000 a year to essentially act like waitstaff at a restaurant, performing services that could be done equally well by far less expensive staff. More importantly, their training and expertise is not utilized effectively because there is a disconnect between the administrators, who actually run the clinic, and the physicians, who are seeing and caring for the patients that visit.

There are many other sources of waste and inefficiency. The large group of patients waiting—often 30-60 minutes—for x-rays could, in many instances, have their images done in the clinic by the doctor using a mini C-arm fluoroscopy unit. These units cost about $60,000 (compared to $200,000 for a regular x-ray unit) and do not require an x-ray technician. They produce excellent images and allow the physician to obtain the ideal view of what he or she is interested in. They save time and money and were standard in every orthopaedic office I had been in until I returned to Canada.

It may seem from this description that the physicians are being short-changed and forced to work in inefficient clinics. On one level, this is true and is a source of frustration for many physicians. However, it is actually the hospital—and by extension, the health system—that is getting a raw deal. Yes, it is frustrating working in a dysfunctional clinic, knowing that if basic principles of clinic organization were employed efficiently, then at least 25% more patients could be seen. However, the reality is that the clinic space is provided free of charge to the physicians. Physicians can, and do, see any patients they want to in the clinic. Physicians are more or less free to decide which patients they will see, when they will see them, and how many patients they will see each day.

They can push their own personal practice's agendas, irrespective of the goals of the hospital and the health system.

Problems treated in the hospital's surgical outpatient department (OPD) include foot and ankle patients, but not spine problems; hand and wrist problems, but not complex hip problems; endocrine surgical problems, but not thoracic surgery problems; complex colon problems, but not liver transplant patients. The hospital's stated mission is to provide expertise in six areas. Yet none of the surgical problems the hospital is treating in its surgical OPD are directly related to those six areas of emphasis. With the exception of cardiac and renal surgery, the surgical conditions emphasized at the hospital, including the surgical OPD, seem to have stemmed from the whims of the involved surgeons, rather than from any clear strategic plan.

The inefficient use of expensive health system resources is only one of many ways that the health system wastes large amounts of money each year. Perhaps the thing that surprised me most when I returned to the Canadian healthcare system was the extent of financial waste. I expected to see a tightly budgeted system that ran lean, but instead I saw waste and financial inefficiency everywhere. Physicians, nurses, administrators, and other healthcare workers were often either underutilized or simply not necessary for the provision of efficient patient care. Tremendous inefficiencies in the use of high-cost resources, such as hospital beds, were the norm. I encountered a general lack of oversight of cost centres for high-cost resources, such as surgical implants. Physicians often received additional payments in the form of poorly-monitored stipends not tied to specific roles or performance standards. Finally, there was little financial transparency.

Canada spends $6,045 per person each year on healthcare[4]—more money per capita than the United Kingdom, Germany, France, Sweden, Australia, and New Zealand.[5] Healthcare expenditures represent

---

[4]   http://www.cihi.ca/web/resource/en/nhex_2014_pubsum_en.pdf

[5]   The Commonwealth Fund: *Mirror, Mirror on the Wall, 2014 Update: How the U.S. Health Care System Compares Internationally.* Karen Davis, Kristof Stremikis, David Squires, Cathy Schoen. Published June 16th 2014: http://www.commonwealthfund.org/publications/fund-reports/2014/jun/mirror-mirror

between 38-42% of the provincial budgets, and in total, 24% of every tax dollar collected in Canada goes toward funding the health system.[6] Despite this cost to taxpayers prescription medications, non-physician services performed outside of a hospital (ex. physiotherapy), essential supplies (ex. crutches, braces, etc.), and most long-term care is *not* covered under the existing Canadian healthcare system. Patients need to pay these expenses themselves. Furthermore, healthcare costs rose 53% between 2004 and 2014—a greater increase than other expenses such as shelter (40.7%), food (15.6%), and clothing (33.4%). Healthcare in Canada is anything but free, and it's getting proportionately more expensive every year.

The Not So Good: Poor-Quality Healthcare

Wrong-sided Surgery

A year before I returned to Canada, one of my future colleagues performed surgery on the wrong leg of a patient. Wrong-sided surgery is a "never event" in medicine—something that should *never* happen.

Six months after I started work, another colleague took a patient to the operating room for an elective bunion surgery. The patient was taken into the room and positioned on the operating table. The leg was prepped and the surgical "timeout" performed. The nurse handed the surgeon a scalpel. He was about to perform surgery on the wrong foot. Fortunately, before he made an incision, he questioned why this patient did not have a bunion deformity. Most bunions occur bilaterally, but fortunately for this patient, the deformity only affected one of her feet. After checking his notes, he realized the mistake. The other leg was prepared, and the surgery was carried out without any other problems.

What happened after this event? Nothing! There was no incident report. There was no team debrief to deconstruct the near-miss. There was no analysis by the nursing, anesthesia, or even my orthopaedic

---

[6]   Milagros Palacios, Bacchus Barua. *The Price of Public Health Care Insurance.* Fraser Research Bulletin. July 2014. http://www.fraserinstitute.org/uploadedFiles/fraser-ca/Content/research-news/research/publications/price-of-public-health-care-insurance-2014.pdf

department. Nothing came out of this incident to minimize the likelihood that this type of event would occur again. After I heard of this episode, I tried to meet with leaders from nursing and anesthesia. It was difficult to arrange a meeting. We exchanged emails, and months went by. It wasn't that these leaders were not interested in what had happened; this was simply not part of their jurisdiction. It was really no one's jurisdiction.

I witnessed the damming effects of a siloed healthcare system—a system based on archaic departmental roles, not on normal patient flows. The system was organized to provide fragmented care, with no group responsible for the overall care that was delivered and the associated results. Furthermore, meaningful outcome data was almost completely absent. How did patients actually do after their treatment? How satisfied were they with their experience? How much did their care cost? No one knew, and no one was held accountable. The end result was medical and surgical care that consistently struggled to be mediocre.

In the case of the wrong-sided surgery "near miss", we were lucky, but there are many other instances where patients are less fortunate. Canadian patients regularly suffer from the care they receive—or the care they fail to receive in a timely manner. As Chapter 3 will outline, patients suffer complications and die at an unacceptably high rate—not because of the individuals working within the system, but because of the way in which the system itself is organized.

Canadians' View of Their Medical System

Canadians, myself included, are strongly supportive of a national, publicly-funded healthcare system. In a 2005 public opinion poll, 87% of those surveyed viewed "eliminating public healthcare" as a negative, believing it would "fundamentally change the nature of Canada."[7,8]

Prior to 2004, many Canadians believed that most problems related to the Canadian healthcare system were largely due to poor

---

[7] Environics & CROP, for CRIC, Portraits of Canada, 2005 (N=~3200)

[8] Soroka, Stuart N. A report to the Health Council of Canada: Canadian Perceptions of the Health Care System. February 2007. http://www.queensu.ca/cora/ files/PublicPerceptions.pdf

management and the government underfunding the system. Based on 2002-2006 data, the Health Council of Canada sponsored a report called "Canadian Perceptions of the Healthcare System". One of the primary conclusions of the report was:

> *"There is overwhelming support for increased spending on healthcare, from both levels of government. There is a strong sense that the federal government should transfer more money to the provinces, but not without conditions—there is also strong support for national standards in healthcare provision."*[9]

To address the perception that healthcare is underfunded, the federal government introduced the Canada Health Transfer (CHT) in 2004. This initiative represented a 10-year commitment to substantially increase the federal government's funding of healthcare. Federal healthcare transfer payments to the provinces increased an average of 6% per year, as an additional $41 billion flowed into the system. Now after 10 years of this increase in funding, with relatively little impact on wait times and quality outcomes, many Canadians question this assumption—especially when they take a closer look at the amount of their taxes devoted to healthcare resources.

Witnessing the healthcare system up close, I found myself asking, "Why aren't Canadians outraged?" They are paying enormous sums of money and receiving mediocre care at best. I noted a "healthcare curtain" that shields the average Canadian (and most healthcare administrators) from observing what is actually happening within their healthcare system. If they had seen but a fraction of what I witnessed, they would likely be appalled.

On July 6th 2013, Asiana Flight 214 crashed while attempting to land at San Francisco International Airport.[10] Three people were killed and 12 passengers critically injured. The accident was front-page news. The Federal Aviation Administration (FAA) in the United States

---

[9]   Soroka, Stuart N. A report to the Health Council of Canada: Canadian Perceptions of the Health Care System. P. 3, February 2007

[10]   http://en.wikipedia.org/wiki/Asiana_Airlines_Flight_214

stepped in quickly to oversee the situation. They issued daily reports and kept the public informed. Quickly, we found out that a commercial pilot in training had been attempting to land the plane, and neither he nor any of the other pilots in the cockpit realized the plane's speed was too low until it was too late. We also found out that one of the rescue fire trucks had tragically run over and killed one of the passengers—a young girl. Subsequent recommendations were forthcoming. The end result was a clear understanding of what had caused this terrible tragedy, and widespread dissemination of the information to minimize the risk of a similar event ever happening again.

For two weeks, the Asiana Airlines crash was prominent in the news. During this same two-week period, an estimated 169—and perhaps as many as 865—Canadians died directly or indirectly from the care (or lack thereof) they received from their healthcare system. Many more suffered unnecessary complications.[11,12] These tragedies were not exciting enough to make the news. If they had been, the headlines may have looked like these:

Sick elderly man admitted to hospital, contracts flu from an unvaccinated healthcare worker, dies a week later in the intensive care unit: cause of death listed as heart failure.

Poor sterile technique during surgery leads to leg infection in a 40-year-old: loses his job as a labourer, becomes depressed, marriage fails.

With some rare, dramatic exceptions, the complications associated with medical care are not newsworthy. They do not make headlines, and therefore do not create a societal impetus for change. It is much easier to maintain an idealized view of the healthcare system than it is to do the hard work that Canadian society and their representative federal and provincial governments need to do in order to effectively reform the system.

---

[11] To Err is Human: Building a Safer Health System. The Institute of Medicine 1999

[12] http://www.alive.com/articles/view/19779/modern_medicine_can_kill

The Healthcare Curtain

At least three components to this figurative curtain prevent the average Canadian from understanding their healthcare system. First, the vast majority of Canadians have limited interaction with the medical system during any given year. Perhaps they see their family doctor, if they are fortunate enough to have one, for a routine exam. Maybe they have an ankle sprain treated in the local emergency room. While important, these are not major interactions with the medical system. It is only when patients really need the healthcare system—when they develop cancer or need to go undergo a major surgery—that they see what the system is really like. Sometimes the stars align and the patient has a good experience. But often they encounter a dysfunctional system characterized by long waits, inconsistent care, and no measurements of the results achieved.

The second element of the healthcare curtain is that Canadians do not have a frame of reference for assessing the quality, efficiency, and cost-effectiveness of their system. In other words, they have nothing to compare it to. Many Canadians believe it is normal to wait six months for surgery. They accept that it is normal to have little or no choice as to where, and from whom, they receive care. They see an absence of coordination between their primary care doctors and their specialists, as well as among other elements within the system, and they come to believe this is "just the way it has to be".

Finally, a superficial view of the healthcare system, such as walking through an outpatient surgical clinic at my former hospital, suggests to the outsider that the system is working, but a deeper view from inside demonstrates the extent of dysfunction.

General Model of the Existing Canadian Healthcare System

Imagine running a business out of a building built in the 1950s. When the building was new, it may have worked well for the business, but over time the nature of the business changed. Gradually over the years, these changes became dramatic, and now the building is completely outdated regarding the present goals of the business it contains.

This is analogous to the structural problem plaguing the various manifestations of the present-day Canadian healthcare system. There is some variation in how the medical system is organized from province to province, but the basic tenets remain the same. Structural processes— that date back more than a half a century to the time of the Canadian healthcare system's birth—have become cemented in place: bulk/yearly funding of hospitals irrespective of performance; physicians that are compensated in isolation from the care that needs to be delivered; siloed departmental structures that preclude coordinated, team-based care delivery; and no meaningful way to ensure accountability of money or quality.

Funding is the lifeblood of the healthcare system. Hospitals are typically funded via bulk/yearly grants, whereas most physicians are paid "fee-for-service" via a separate pile of money that is disconnected from hospital funding. The hospital I worked at was fairly typical. Each year, they received close to $700 million in funds, usually with about a 2-4% yearly increase to account for inflation. Hospitals are essentially paid regardless of productivity or outcomes. Upon receiving the money, the hospital allocates it to the various programs and departments to carry out their respective tasks. At this point, the bloated paper bureaucracy takes over. There is a seemingly endless supply of middle managers, who are disconnected from the playing field that control the funding. Departments of Medicine, Nursing, Surgery, and Housecleaning typically all function in isolation.

Quality of care is undermined because established principles of high value healthcare delivery cannot be effectively instituted.[13] It is difficult or impossible to establish physician-led teams that focus on the ultimate outcome of care, work in a coordinated manner, and continuously improve the process based on the results they achieve. Instead, fee-for service funding dictates that individual physicians interface with this system in isolated and idiosyncratic ways. In most instances they function as private business owners working in support of their own agendas.

---

[13] *Value* in healthcare has been defined by Michael Porter as "health outcomes achieved per dollar spent." Porter M. What is value in health care. *N Eng J Med* 2010; 363: 2477-2481.

The system as a whole has a distinct lack of focus on outputs—patients seen and care provided. This is combined with an entrenched organization structure built on a defective foundation and encumbered by countless failed *work arounds*. The resulting system resists change, precisely at a time when flexibility and creativity in system organization is demanded. This organizational structure may have worked well 50 years ago. At that time, care for most major illnesses and surgeries was provided in hospitals by physicians who worked largely in isolation. In the modern age of medicine—where care must be team-based, outcomes are paramount, and organizational flexibility is essential—this organizational structure fails. The end result is a discombobulated system with patients and taxpayers suffering.

Summary

Let's return to the interview with our hypothetical professional hockey team. From a hockey point of view, it is ludicrous to organize a professional team in this manner and expect to be successful. However, this is analogous to how much of the Canadian healthcare system is organized.

The owners are the various provincial governments. They hire nice people and give large bulk funding to hospital and health authorities each year, essentially irrespective of performance. Yes, they do make changes on occasion, but these are invariably only tweaks around the edges—changes that do not fundamentally demand excellence or performance in terms of taking care of the patients or the population.

The general manager represents the hospital administrators, a large team of individuals who are almost always completely disconnected from the healthcare playing field. They control funding and organize care—as it has always been organized. They study reams of data of questionable accuracy and attend countless meetings. In many instances, administrators are "gamed" by doctors, nurses, and others working in the system.

From an organizational point of view, there is no head coach—no individual who is ultimately responsible for each patient's episode of care. Who is looking after the patient and assessing the results of care? The answer is typically "no one". Why? Simply put, the system is siloed—organized around isolated departments. It's not oriented around *episodes of care* or *programs* to provide care to specific patient populations—what is known as a *service line* approach. It has always been this way, and there is no sign this structure will change any time soon.

Akin to having multiple assistant coaches with no head coach, every group looks after their own best interests. The Operating Room (OR) Nursing Department looks after the OR nurses. The ward nurses look after the ward nurses. The anesthesiologists look after the anesthesiologists. The surgeons look after the surgeons. And the administrators look after the administrators. Yet the system is organized so that no one is truly looking after the patients' best interests.

The hockey player, happy with his game despite the team losing 6-0, is representative of most healthcare providers. This should in no way imply that they are happy when patients receive a suboptimal outcome. Rather, it is a simple reality that in most instances they never know what the final "outcome" is, and their compensation and wellbeing are not tied to patient outcomes. Compensation is instead tied to other aspects. Nurses and other employees are rewarded for simply showing up. Physicians are rewarded for seeing a high volume of patients. In some instances, compensation is unintentionally structured to reward poor patient care.

Mindless bulk funding on a yearly basis with no accountability for outcomes. Management that is completely disconnected from the playing field. No single individual clearly leading the team. And individual players functioning in their own best interests. This is no way to run a professional hockey team, and it is no way to run a modern healthcare system.

Summary Points: Chapter 1

- Canadians are strongly supportive of the concept of a national, publicly funded healthcare system that provides high-quality care to all citizens. However, evidence increasingly demonstrates that the current system falls far short of these goals.

- The organizational structure of the Canadian healthcare system is based on history—not on normal patient flows. Fragmented care delivery is the norm, often with no group responsible for the overall results of care. This predictably leads to quality of care that is suboptimal and costs that are expensive, the details of which are discussed in Chapters 2 and 3.

- A figurative *healthcare curtain* prevents the average Canadian from seeing and truly understanding their healthcare system.

- The system as a whole has a distinct lack of focus on outputs—patients seen and care provided. This is combined with an entrenched organization structure built on a defective foundation and encumbered by countless failed *work arounds*. The resulting system resists change, precisely at a time when system organization demands flexibility and creativity.

CHAPTER 2

Expensive Medical Care

How would a professional hockey team approach the following financial situations?

Jerry Norman is an aging player in his late 30s. He has a contract that is up for renewal. Five years ago, he was one of the team's stars, but now his skills have declined with age. He still brings effort to the arena every day, but he is demanding a high-priced contract over a number of years.

Three years ago, Bobby James was highly touted. He was drafted fourth overall in the first round. Since then, he has struggled. His first year, he failed to make the team and had to return to junior hockey. In his second year, he made the team but has fluctuated between the third and fourth line. His potential has been unfulfilled to date. More concerning, he has developed a reputation as being petulant and lazy. His contract is up for renewal, and he has demanded to be paid an amount equivalent to those in his draft class that are now stars.

Fred Johnson is a 27-year-old defenseman who has been with the team for two years after spending five years in the minor leagues. He is not a flashy player, scoring only five goals and 21 assists last year. However, he has emerged as a solid defender, who is often asked to kill penalties and line up against the opposing teams' best players. He is quiet, but the coaches feel he may be the hardest-working player on the team. He is becoming a role model for younger players. He has been paid the league minimum for the past two years. He is requesting a fair contract.

Introduction: Story of the Surgical Implants

"Your department is spending a lot of money on surgical implants," the administrator in charge of finances for the hospital's surgical program told me. "How much?" I inquired. "I am not exactly sure," she said, "but it's a lot." I had been expecting this conversation for over a year. It was actually a conversation I attempted to initiate six months earlier. Many surgical operations require implants: plates and screws to fix fractures, joint replacements to replace arthritic joints, and a variety of other "implants" that are inserted into the body in order to achieve the desired results of surgery. Implant manufacturing is a huge business, and implants in general are very expensive—often more than $1000 per operation, though the prices are widely variable.

Large organizations can often achieve dramatic price reductions by ensuring that surgeons use the lowest-cost implant when choosing between equivalent implants—or by instituting simple negotiation techniques. This did happen at the provincial and regional level for common items, such as joint replacements, with excellent price reductions. However, for most of the orthopaedic implants used at our hospital, there was little or no discussion about cost.

Given the cost, I had expected that administrators would have had a much greater interest in the overall expense of implants. However, there was a distinct lack of oversight of this cost centre—and many other equivalent cost centres. Illustrative of this problem was a complete disconnect between the surgeons, who were implanting these orthopaedic devices, and the administrators, who were paying for them. The surgeons had no idea how much the implants cost, and the administrators had no idea how the implants they were paying for were being used.

Imagine a restaurant ordering food and supplies, cooking meals, and then paying for these supplies. Now imagine that the individuals ordering the food were completely disconnected from the chefs who cooked the food, and they in turn were disconnected from those paying for it. Any business selling to this restaurant that realized this organizational structure existed would likely elevate their prices significantly. This is essentially what the companies selling orthopaedic implants to the hospitals do.

This was not an isolated episode, and the lack of oversight of cost centres with high-cost resources seemed to be the norm. Other forms of financial inefficiency are even more problematic. Financial inefficiency within the Canadian healthcare system takes many forms, including:

1. Bulk funding of hospital services
2. A dysfunctional physician compensation model
3. A general lack of financial transparency
4. Poor allocation of human resources
5. Inefficient use of hospital bed resources
6. Poor monitoring of performance-based payments

Big Picture View: The Cost of the Canadian Healthcare System—Anything but "Free"

When I returned to Canada in 2010, I expected to find a healthcare system running lean. I knew there were long waits for many surgeries, and access to care was a challenge. I assumed erroneously that this was due to a lack of resources. During my time working within the Canadian healthcare system, nothing surprised me more than the extent of financial inefficiency I witnessed on a day-to-day basis. The problem with the healthcare system was not a lack of funds. The problem was how these funds were used. There were reoccurring themes of waste and inefficiency. All of these themes seemed to stem directly, or indirectly, from the manner in which the system itself was organized.

It is estimated that in 2013 Canadians spent a total of $211 billion on healthcare. Of this amount, taxpayers contributed 70.1% ($148 billion) via the federal or provincial governments.[14] This represents the public funding of healthcare—24.4% of every tax dollar collected in Canada.[15] The per capita cost in 2012 was $4,602. This equates to 10.6% of the

---

[14] Canadian Institute for Health Information [CIHI] (2013). National Health Expenditure Trends, 1975-2013. Canadian Institute for Health Information. P. viii. https://secure.cihi.ca/free_products/NHEXTrendsReport_EN.pdf (accessed April 4th 2015)

[15] Palacios M, Bacchus B. The Price of Public Health Care Insurance. Fraser Research Bulletin July 2014. P. 7

Gross Domestic Product (GDP).[16] This was greater than per capita healthcare costs in most other developed nations including: the United Kingdom, France, Germany, Australia, New Zealand, and Sweden.[17]

As the above figures demonstrate, 30% of healthcare costs are borne by private citizens, above and beyond the taxes they pay. The various provincial Medicare programs only cover "medical necessary" care and physician payments.[18] Medications, physiotherapy, nursing homes, durable medical equipment such as braces, orthotics, and crutches—even money that some patients choose to spend on jumping the often-excessively long queue for treatment—are all part of this substantial, additional, "non tax" cost. The reality is that healthcare in Canada is actually quite expensive despite the widely held public perception to the contrary.

Funding and administration of healthcare is the responsibility of each provincial government, albeit with large federal transfer payments helping to support each provincial health system. In the past decade, healthcare budgets have consumed an increasing percentage of provincial (and federal) budgets to the detriment of other essential government services, such as education, transportation, and the environment. From 2000 to 2012, total healthcare spending in Canada more than doubled—from under $100 billion to $205.4 billion.[19] From 2004 to 2014, healthcare costs increased 53.3%, compared to an 18.7% increase in the consumer price index. This rate of increase in healthcare expenditures far outpaced other costs, such as food, clothing, and shelter.[20] Provincial

---

[16]   Figures from the Organization for Economic Co-operation and Development (OECD) as reported in *The Globe and Mail*. October 31, 2014 p A8.

[17]   Karen Davis, Kristof Stremikis, David Squires, and Cathy Schoen. Mirror, Mirror on the Wall: Performance of the U.S. Health Care System Compares Internationally. The Commonwealth Fund. p.7. June 2014

[18]   Canada Health Act: Frequently Asked Questions. http://www.hc-sc.gc.ca/hcs-sss/medi-assur/faq-eng.php (accessed January 17th, 2016)

[19]   National Health Expenditure Trends: 1975-2014. Canadian Institute for Health information. October 2014. p 20. http://www.cihi.ca/web/resource/en/nhex_2014_report_en.pdf

[20]   Palacios M, Bacchus B. The Price of Public Health Care Insurance. Fraser Research Bulletin July 2014. P. 6

healthcare spending increased almost 7% annually from 2000 to 2010, and as of 2015, healthcare averages 42% of the provincial budgets.[21]

This rate of growth creates an excessive strain on provincial budgets, and recent budgets have seen a leveling-off of the rate of healthcare spending. Nevertheless, with an appetite to spend and an aging population requiring more medical care, the pressure to funnel increasing amounts of each provincial budget into healthcare will be great. This has led many to question the long-term sustainability of the existing healthcare system.[22]

"*Price is what you pay. Value is what you get.*"[23] Paying a great deal for healthcare might be acceptable if the care was outstanding, access was readily available, and financial inefficiencies were minimal—i.e., if the system provided high *value* healthcare. As will be outlined in this chapter and the next, major deficits in each of these areas are common in the existing Canadian healthcare system. It seems fundamental healthcare reform is inevitable; it is just a matter of when—and how.

Sources of Financial Inefficiency in the Canadian Healthcare System

So what has led to poor financial performance within the healthcare system? Let's review the aforementioned six recurring themes.

1. Bulk Funding of Hospital Services: just "keep the lights on" and wait for March madness

For 11 months of the year at my hospital, money was tight. Unless it had been budgeted more than a year in advance, there was no opportunity to add new staff, new equipment, or innovative new programs. All the

---

21 http://www.theglobeandmail.com/news/national/health-care-spending-projected-to-grow-at-slowest-pace-in-17-years/article21384941/

22 Sustainability of the Canadian Healthcare System and Impact of the 2014 Revision of the Canada Health Transfer. Canadian Institute of Actuaries and Society of Actuaries. September 2013

23 Quote attributed to Warren Buffett

while, outdated existing programs, and individuals whose jobs seemed to have no clear purpose, persisted—ensconced in the existing system. Then the month of March rolled around, and a stream of money was released into the system. Actually, it was usually late January when we would hear about "extra funds", but by the end of March, these funds needed to be spent.

The reason for this March madness was simple. March 31st was the end of the hospital's fiscal year. In the weeks leading up to the March 31st deadline, individual physicians, department chairs, and administrators would argue about how this money should be spent. Emails were exchanged. Meetings were had. Orthopaedics wanted a new mini C-arm fluoroscopy unit for their outpatient clinic. The general surgeons wanted a new portable ultrasound unit for their breast surgeries. The ophthalmologist wanted a new YAG laser. More than 100 requests for new equipment were entertained. Most of these requests could not be filled. However, the opportunity for even some financial windfall was enough to send everyone into a feeding frenzy. Then on March 31, it was all over. The extra piles of money that the administrators had been hiding for a rainy day had been spent. It was back to the stagnant way of funding care. This was one of the quirks of bulk funding of healthcare, also known as *global budgeting*—lump sums provided to individual hospitals to cover their operating expenses for a fixed period of time.[24]

Administrators needed to spend all of the money they were allocated and not a penny more. Having a surplus just meant returning the money back to whence it came—and potentially not getting as much the following year.

Bulk funding of hospital services from the provincial governments, either directly or indirectly, is the primary means by which most healthcare in Canada is funded, whereas in other healthcare systems, funding is directly or indirectly tied to productivity and performance. Canada's use of bulk funding is unique. It is the predominant source of funding for hospital services, and practically speaking, there are

---

[24] Sutherland JM, Crump RT, Repin N, Hellsten E. Paying for Hospital Services: A Hard Look at the Options. *CD Howe Institute, Commentary 378.* April 2013. P. 3

few, if any, strings attached to receiving the money. As one of my colleagues said, "All the hospital needs to do to get their money is keep the lights on."

Jason Sutherland, Associate Professor at the University of British Columbia's Centre for Health Services and Policy Research has outlined the limitations of global budgeting.[25] Collectively, these limitations have a profoundly negative effect on how healthcare is delivered in Canada. Transparency is very difficult with bulk funding. It is hard or impossible to determine whether two hospitals are providing equivalent care for the money they are receiving. In addition, historical inefficiencies are perpetuated by global budgeting. They create a sense of entitlement, whereby hospitals expect to get funding year after year for doing what they had previously done. Why change the culture when it won't lead to increased funding, and may in fact be quite disruptive to the way of doing business that everyone is used to?

Professor Sutherland and others have argued that global budgeting has an adverse effect on access to elective surgery. He also argues that it contributes to the persistence of large, unexplained variations in both utilization and cost of care. Bulk funding of healthcare stifles innovation, as this form of payment removes a major incentive to introduce fundamental changes in care delivery that could substantially improve care and/or decrease cost. This means that new practices that reduce lengths of stays or other drivers of health cost are not likely to be introduced. It also means that the penalties for inefficiencies are minimal or non-existent.

2. A Dysfunctional Physician Compensation Model: the rich surgical resident

When I was an orthopaedic resident in the mid 1990s, one of my surgical-resident colleagues was named Johnny. Johnny was a well-liked, outgoing, high-energy, multilingual Ear, Nose, and Throat (ENT) resident.

---

[25]   Jason Sutherland. Hospital payment mechanisms: options for Canada (Presentation). Centre for Health Services Research Foundation (CHSRF): Healthcare financing, innovation and transformation. Ottawa, March 18, 2011.

One year in early April, a few of my surgical resident colleagues were looking through the "Blue Book"—the British Columbia Ministry of Health's financial statement for the Medical Services Commission (MSC). It listed how much money every doctor in the province had collected from the provincial government during the previous fiscal year. After reviewing the billings of some of the prominent surgeons who were teaching us, one of the residents said, "Check out Johnny's billings." I did not know what he meant. We were all hard-working surgical residents with barely enough time to have any sort of a life outside of the hospital. How could a surgical resident make any kind of money billing the medical system? However, when they checked Johnny's billings for the previous year, it was $141,254.

It turned out that Johnny worked at a small clinic for six hours every Saturday that he was not on call. He would regularly see 80-100 patents during that time, spending a couple of minutes with each patient, often writing them prescriptions for vitamins or other placebo-type medications. He was quite open about his job, saying that although he did not practice much "real medicine", the patients were grateful to be able to chat with a doctor in their native language.

The province of British Columbia has since put limits on the number of new patients a physician can see in a day, in order to try to curtail this type of activity—and residents are no longer eligible for an unrestricted medical license until they graduate. However, this *churn and burn* (i.e., race through a busy clinic) mentality not only still exists, it seems to be predominant. After all, in a fee-for-service compensation model, it makes a great deal of financial sense for a doctor if he or she can practice this way. This payment model rewards volume; seeing more patients means making more money.

My present orthopaedic practice in San Francisco is largely a fee-for-service practice. I get paid for each patient I see in the office, and each surgery I perform. The more patients I see, the more money I collect. However, there are a finite number of patients in my community, and quite a few physicians. Patients will simply go elsewhere if they do not get the service or results they expect. If I started cutting corners with patients (e.g., taking limited time to see and examine them, not answering their questions adequately, or racing through surgeries at the expense of quality), I would quickly find myself with a shortage of patients. This rarely ever happens in Canada. The restriction on physician job openings means the supply of patients usually exceeds the capacity of practicing physicians.

One of the dirty secrets of the fee-for-service Canadian healthcare system is that the worse you are as a physician, the more money you are likely to make. While this axiom is not always true, it is true much more often than not. In a fee-for-service system with high patient demand (i.e., an abundance of patients who want to be seen), the less time a physician spends with each patient + the less detailed the physical examination they perform + the less time they take in explaining treatment options to patients = the more patients they see, and the more money they will make!

It is not a subtle difference either; see twice as many patients, and you make twice as much money—actually more, given that most practice expenses are fixed. In a pure fee-for-service model with an oversupply of patients, there is very strong financial pressure for physicians to cut corners. Fee-for-service compensation does not pay for quality; it in fact serves as a financial disincentive to practice high-quality, patient-centred medicine.

In February 2014, Russ Jones, the Auditor General of British Columbia, released his report on the oversight of physician services.[26] He highlighted the lack of monitoring of performance-based payments for physicians as being a core problem with the healthcare system. He pointed out that payments are generally not tied to quality, so governments cannot demonstrate that physician services are high-quality. Neither are payments tied to cost-effectiveness. In addition, he noted that, *"Physicians can only charge for services that they perform themselves. This restricts physicians from working in interdisciplinary teams, which have been shown to improve patient satisfaction, access, and equity."* He concluded that governments cannot demonstrate that compensation for physician services is cost-effective.

What I saw in my two years within the Canadian healthcare system stunned me. The BC Auditor General and the citizens of Canada are

---

[26] Jones R. *Oversight of Physician Services*. Office of the Auditor General of British Columbia. February 2014.

right to be concerned about the value they are receiving from their physicians.

3. Lack of Financial Transparency: the disappearing $2.1 million

During the 2011 fiscal year, the hospital I work at received $2.1 million in Activity-Based Funding (ABF). ABF has been described as a generic term encompassing a variety of funding methods designed to fund health systems, hospitals, or providers based on the types and volume of patients they treat.[27,28] ABF which includes *Diagnostic Related Group (DRG)-based funding, Payments by Results, Pay for Performance,* and *Patient Focused Funding,* is a strategy to help ensure a health system is paying for healthcare services it needs—i.e., paying for value. Some form of direct or indirect ABF, is the predominant means of healthcare funding throughout the world.

However, it was only recently introduced to Canada when British Columbia started a specific type of ABF program in 2009.[29] The program designated a relatively small percentage (~4%) of the BC provincial healthcare budget to fund specific healthcare "activities". ABF differs markedly from the traditional *global budgeting* approach to funding healthcare in Canada, which provides bulk yearly funding to the system—and then hopes enough care is delivered. The idea behind the British Columbia version of ABF was to purchase specific healthcare services to address demand that was not being met by the existing system.

In British Columbia, one of the areas that had high-patient demand was foot and ankle and upper-extremity care—exactly the type of care my colleagues and I provided. My hospital applied for and received ABF money, specifically to increase the volume of foot and hand patients seen

---

27 Sutherland JM, Crump RT, Repin N, Hellsten E. Paying for Hospital Services: A Hard Look at the Options. *CD Howe Institute, Commentary 378.* April 2013. P. 5

28 http://healthcarefunding.ca/key-issues/activity-based-funding/

29 Hospital Funding Policy and Activity-Based Funding. EvidenceNetwork.ca http://umanitoba.ca/outreach/evidencenetwork/costs-and-spending/costs7

and treated. The $2.1 million in additional funding was received by the hospital—and then proceeded to disappear into the system.

The physicians actually treating these patients with foot and hand conditions had no oversight of this money. We had no input and were not consulted as to how it might be best spent to improve productivity. Eventually, I received a budgeted breakdown of where the money was purportedly being spent: extra clinic nurses that were not needed; anesthesia care that was already being paid for through the provincial medical services plan; and extra orthopaedic operating time which—if we did receive it—was certainly not earmarked specifically for foot and hand surgery cases, but rather spread among all the areas within orthopaedics. The money was essentially funneled directly into the regular hospital budget, completely undermining the intended goals of the ABF program.

Lack of financial transparency and lack of input from clinicians are recurring themes and fundamental problems within the health system. There was a near complete disconnect between those making decisions as to how money would be spent and those individuals actually taking care of patients. Lack of clinician input into hospital budgeting was one of the most surprising and disappointing features I observed within the Canadian healthcare system. When I took the position as head of the department of orthopaedics, it never occurred to me to ask whether I would have oversight of the orthopaedic-related budget. At the previous institutions where I had worked in the United States, the leader of the orthopaedic department always had oversight of the orthopaedic-related budget—albeit working closely with a hospital administrator. Furthermore, department heads would be held responsible for the financial performance of their service line. More than a few orthopaedic department chairs have lost their jobs due to underperformance in the financial arena. Recent initiatives such as British Columbia's Facility Based Physician program administered through the Specialists Services Committee (SSC) have attempted to address this issue in a rudimentary manner.[30] However, the predominant paradigm remains

---

[30]   http://sscbc.ca/partnership-work/supporting-facility-based-physicians

one of disconnecting the finances of the health system from those individuals who are delivering care.

The need to have clinician leaders directly involved in budgeting was obvious. They know the care that needs to be delivered to the patients they are treating. Physicians who are providing direct patient care are usually in the best position to determine what resources are necessary to deliver this care, identify and eliminate waste, propose effective cost-reduction strategies, and most effectively prioritize the allocation of funds. The system I observed in Canada not only did not seek clinician input on a regular basis, it seemed to actively hide the finances from those providing medical care—those best positioned to determine how the money should be most effectively spent.

4. Poor Allocation of Human Resources: staffing the surgical outpatient clinic

Every day that I saw patients in the hospital's surgical outpatient clinic, I had a registered nurse (RN) assigned to work with me. It was usually one of three or four nurses, but I never knew who it would be until I arrived at the clinic that day. The nurses were nice and friendly. They performed a series of basic tasks, such as getting patients from the waiting room, taking off dressings, and giving patients handouts. They tried to be helpful, and on a basic level, they were. Furthermore, they did not cost me a penny. They were fully paid for by the hospital out of the surgical program budget, and thus, "free" to the physicians.

A closer examination of the work these nurses did would lead to the quick realization that a medical assistant (MA) or licensed practical nurse (LPN), whose salary was 25% less, could easily perform these services.[31] If the surgeons whose patients were being cared for were responsible for the costs incurred, this registered nurse would function quite differently. The nurse would be used "to the level of their license". They would see patients independently and would help with the throughput of patients. But that was not how the system was organized. Instead, administrators disconnected from the delivery of care decided in a seemingly arbitrary

---

[31] An LPN in Vancouver BC makes an average of $24.96/hour versus an RN who makes an average of $31.00. www.payscale.com (accessed November 15th 2015)

manner who would work and what they would be doing. The end result was that these individuals were severely underutilized.

Dysfunctional allocation of human resources is one of the primary sources of financial waste within the healthcare system. Various healthcare providers, such as nurses and physical therapists, are hired by the hospital. However, without specific, clinician-led service lines or teams oriented to deliver specific types of care, these healthcare providers often functioned in an isolated, idiosyncratic, and inefficient manner. Equally problematic examples of dysfunctional allocation of expensive human resources included countless hospital administrators who were not specifically involved in patient care, and whose practical purpose was unclear despite very official-sounding job titles.

5. Inefficient Use of Hospital Bed Resources: the ward's favourite

Mark was a gentle and low-functioning 36-year-old, the child of an alcoholic mother. One September evening he broke his ankle and was admitted to the orthopaedic ward. He never had surgery; he just stayed. He stayed 24 hours—the time it took to control his pain with oral pain medication. He stayed two weeks, at which point his cast was changed. He stayed six weeks, at which point his fracture had healed and he could walk. He stayed three months, six months, nine months. All the while, he took up one of our $700+/day acute beds on the orthopaedic ward.

He was pleasant to have around the ward and required minimal nursing care—just his meals and the charting of his vital signs twice a day. This contrasted with the more intense work required to manage patients recovering from recent surgery. Mark quickly became a ward favourite. Everyone would stop and chat with him. He finally left the orthopaedic ward in July of the following year—ten months after he was admitted.

The story of Mark, "The Ward's Favourite", illustrates the cost of poor resource utilization. Mark's situation is not unique. On average, there were between two and four patients like him on our 24-bed acute orthopaedic ward—and an equivalent percentage on other wards. They have been described as *Alternative Level of Care* (ALC) patients or *orphan patients*[32]—patients who do not require acute care or active medical or surgical management, yet cannot be discharged. The factors preventing their discharge are often psychosocial or administrative. They need minimal care but cannot leave the hospital because they have nowhere to go, or because the resources needed for their discharge have not been marshaled. Of the 450 acute beds at our hospital, a conservative estimate is that at least 50, and probably closer to 100, are taken up by these orphan patients. The end results are higher costs and chronic bed shortages—often leading to acute patients who do need admission remaining backed up in the emergency room, awaiting a bed. Hospitals are simply not held accountable for these sorts of inefficiencies.

Prudent resource management would dictate that discharge-planning resources should be concentrated on these patients, and that those who cannot be discharged be transferred to less expensive care units that provide substantially less expensive nursing support. This was the norm at the previous hospitals I had worked at.

In Canada, about 14% of hospitalized patients have been officially designated as ALC patients.[33] They no longer have an acute medical problem and therefore do not need to be taking up a bed in an acute hospital—yet they do. Each day across the country approximately 7500 hospital beds are filled with these ALC patients. However, the actual number of these orphaned patients is invariably much higher. In order to keep the *official* number of ALC patients down to a reasonable level, some hospitals reengineered how a patient is classified as an ALC patient. Rather than let the treating physician determine when a patient was no longer an acute patient, they introduced a designated individual or team to classify these patients. An "acute patient" would remain an acute patient until they were reclassified—regardless of whether they required active acute treatment—until they were formally designated as an extended-care patient. This process could take an additional week

---

[32]   *Orphan patients* has also been used as a term to describe patients in the health system who do not have their own family physician.

[33]   Sutherland JM, Crump RT. Exploring Alternative Level of Care and the Role of Funding Policies: An Evolving Evidence Base for Canada. Canadian Health Services Research Foundation (CHSRF) Series of Reports on Cost Drivers and Health System Efficiency: Paper 8, September 2011. www.chsrf.ca

or longer, meaning that many patients who should be designated as ALC are not.

ALC patients represent an extraordinary expense to the system, and serve to deprive patients who do need acute hospitalization of the beds and care they need. This situation is particularly frustrating given that a fix (moving patients to substantially less expensive beds) is conceptually straightforward. Unfortunately, waste and inefficiency, as illustrated by dysfunctional bed utilizations, seemed to be built into the system. Furthermore, there was no real impetus for change, so the problems remained year after year, decade after decade. Having seen a different system tackle this type of problem in an efficient and effective manner, it was painful to watch the waste.

6. Inadequate Monitoring of Performance-Based Payments: "shut-up" money

One of the physicians at my hospital received the equivalent of $50,000 per year from the hospital. It was widely known that he received this money, but nobody seemed to know why—not even the administrators who were giving it to him. There were no clear deliverables, and the administrators who had set up this annual payment agreement were now gone. Still, the payments continued. It was seemingly easier to persist with this outflow of money than to ask the hard questions and make the difficult decisions to stop it. This sort of outflow of money without regard for end results seemed to be the norm.

Like other physicians in administrative or pseudo-administrative positions, I received a stipend for my role as head of the orthopaedic department—in my case $100,000 per year. There must have been a job description for what I was to do somewhere, but it was certainly not enforced. I would like to think I worked hard for this money, answering emails and proactively attempting to improve the experience for orthopaedic patients. The reality is that all I needed to do was attend a few committee meetings each month in order to collect this money. Many physicians in these appointed positions did choose to do the minimum, and doing the bare minimum, or even doing the normal amount of work, meant these types of payments were lucrative for physicians.

Fragmented payments for titled positions (Head of this, Assistant Director of that) are the norm. Some of the administrators call these payments "shut up" money—money to buy silence or to keep doctors placated while the administrators run the show. The money flows out, but the services do not flow in. These funds, while individually small, are collectively quite large. Each year, they are ensconced in the budget like a large rock that cannot be moved.

The Root Causes of Financial Dysfunction

These financial inefficiencies, as well as many other inefficiencies that are inherent in the Canadian healthcare system, are usually not the product of individuals acting maliciously. Rather, they are the predictable outcome of the manner in which the system is organized and funded. Fundamentally, the system is organized to pay for inputs, not outputs. By "outputs", I mean the end results of care—patients seen and effectively treated. This is as opposed to "inputs" to the system, such as doctors, nurses, administrators, and equipment—all essential for producing the end product of care. However, paying them in isolation from the end results creates major problems.

Hospitals receive recurring "bulk funding" each year, essentially regardless of their performance. Physicians working in a fee-for-service model get paid for each patient seen, regardless of the outcome of treatment or how well they integrate within the healthcare team. Ensuring the perpetuation of this system is fragmented administrative departments with siloed budgets. Each group protects its own turf, even though amalgamations and reorganizations would be far better for patients and taxpayers. Finally, the lack of financial transparency—and the absence of any external, independent, accurate oversight of healthcare finances—ensures a spectacularly expensive healthcare system.

In my estimation, these financial inefficiencies increase the cost of healthcare—not merely by 2% or 5%, but rather by 30% or more.[34] The potential for saving healthcare dollars, while dramatically improving the quality and timeliness of care, is huge. To achieve this performance improvement, we need a fundamental restructuring of the way the healthcare system itself is organized. The principles underlying how this restructuring can be done are outlined in Chapters 6, 7, and 8. A specific example of how fundamental reformed can be achieved is outlined in Chapter 9.

Summary

There is a great deal that healthcare can learn from how a professional hockey team manages its finances. Each NHL team has to function within a salary cap –a fixed amount they can spend on players established by the league.[35] Fundamentally, a hockey team is looking to pay for results. Funding is not separated from outputs. Each player, coach, and resource is funded, according to their ability or perceived ability, to generate an end result. General managers and team presidents who get this equation correct are rewarded with new contracts. Those who fail are fired. Players who demand too much money, even those who were stars in the past, are not rewarded with lucrative contracts by prudent general managers. Meanwhile, players who bring high value to the team through their work ethic or particular niche skills are given appropriate contracts.

Each team may have a yearly budget, but this is fluid within the constraints of the salary cap; it is not blindly administered based on

---

[34] To illustrate the potential savings a comparison to the United Kingdom's healthcare system is warranted. According to the 2014 Commonwealth report per capital healthcare costs are 32% less in the United Kingdom. Despite this the UK's system rated 1st overall compared to Canada, which rated 10th out of 11 countries.

[35] The NHL has a "hard" (fixed) salary cap. The amount is set each season based on the league's revenue from the previous season. For the 2015-16 season this has been set at $71.4 million. https://en.wikipedia.org/wiki/NHL_salary_cap

what has always been done. There are fixed costs (e.g., salaries that have already been negotiated and the general expenses of running the team), but there is wide flexibility on how the remaining money is spent. Underlying all of this is the knowledge that the team's general manager and president will ultimately be held accountable for the team's performance on the ice.

Finally, there is financial transparency for all to see. The sports writers and the public do not have control of the team's budget, but they can easily view where the money is going. They can, and do, comment on its appropriateness. General managers and team presidents who spend inappropriately, either through poorly-negotiated contracts or money that is spent in unproductive areas, do not find themselves employed for long.

Paying for results, variable budgets that are tightly managed, and full financial transparency are characteristics of the financial organization of a professional hockey team. Canadian healthcare could benefit greatly from a movement towards this type of model.

Summary Points: Chapter 2

- Healthcare in Canada is anything but *free*. In 2014 Canadians spent an estimated $6,045 per person—70% of this was paid from tax revenue via the provincial and federal governments, and an additional 30% was paid out of pocket for health services not covered by the provincial health plans (ex. medications, physical therapy, etc.). This ranked Canada as one of the most expensive healthcare systems in the world.

- Financial inefficiency within the Canadian healthcare system takes many forms, including:

  1. Bulk funding of hospital services
  2. A dysfunctional physician compensation model
  3. A general lack of financial transparency
  4. Poor allocation of human resources
  5. Inefficient use of hospital bed resources
  6. Poor monitoring of performance-based payments

- Bulk funding in the form of yearly lump sum payments is the primary means by which hospitals get funded within the Canadian system. This approach to funding tends to perpetuate the status quo and removes a major incentive to introduce fundamental changes in care delivery that could substantially improve care and/or decrease cost.

- Physicians in Canada are predominantly compensated on a fee-for-service basis. This mode of payment rewards mediocre care in the form of high volume, lower-quality patient interactions, and it discourages working in interdisciplinary teams, which have been shown to improve patient satisfaction, access, and equity.

- Financial inefficiencies in the Canadian healthcare system are the predictable outcome of the manner in which the system is organized and funded. Fundamentally, the system is organized to pay for inputs, not outputs.

CHAPTER 3

Mediocre Healthcare

On January 5th 2015, Dave Nonis, Vice President of Hockey Operations for the Toronto Maple Leafs, fired head coach Randy Carlyle. Carlyle was hired by the Leafs in March of 2012 after having previously coached the Anaheim Ducks—including a Stanley Cup victory in 2007. However, the Leafs failed to excel during his coaching tenure. With the team in 4th place in its division and having lost 7 of their previous 10 games, he was relieved of his job. On April 12th 2015, Nonis and the remaining coaching staff of the Leafs were also fired after the team finished the 2014-15 season 27th in the 30-team NHL.

On November 1st 2011, Washington Capitals star player Alexander Ovechkin was benched during the third period of a close game between his Washington Capitals and the Anaheim Ducks. He desperately wanted to get on the ice, but the team's coach Bruce Boudreau kept him anchored to the bench. Ovechkin had been named one of the NHL's first team All-Stars five years in a row, and he had won the Hart Memorial trophy as the league's most valuable player twice in the previous four years. However, Boudreau was not happy with Ovechkin's effort and performance. He made the decision that sitting Ovechkin on the bench during that critical junction of the third period was the right thing to do for the team as a whole. With Ovechkin on the bench, the Capitals tied the game—and subsequently went on to win in overtime.

In professional hockey, team performance matters. General managers, coaches, and players all know this fact. Decisions, including who should play and how they should play, are all made with the goal of optimizing the team's overall performance. Job security is dependent on overall results.

Canadian Healthcare and Quality: How is the System Really Doing?

For 18-year-old Frankie Jefferson, the day that changed his life forever started like many others—hanging out with his buddies from high school. It was a brilliant, sunny day in August 1992, and Frankie and his friends had converged down by the river that ran through their small town in Northern British Columbia. They were joking, horseplaying, smoking, and drinking—with regular breaks to cool off with a swim in the river.

As the day wore on and the alcohol took hold of their systems, their antics grew more animated. It wasn't long before Frankie and his friends were jumping off the 15-foot-high bridge that spanned the river and contained the main road that headed into town. They had done this before, but no one had ever dived in headfirst—not until Frankie did it that fateful August day. His body sliced through the water, and moments later his head crashed into the bottom of the river.

The water had slowed his speed somewhat, but his head was still driven forward with tremendous force, breaking his neck. He floated to the surface, unable to move his arms and legs. His friends, realizing the gravity of the situation, gently lifted his body and head out of the water so he would not drown. They called the local ambulance. His spine was immobilized, and he was raced off to the regional emergency room in Prince George.

Dr. Fredrickson was working at the emergency room, and after an initial assessment including x-rays, he determined that Frankie had a dislocation of the 5th cervical vertebrae on the 6th with resulting quadriplegia. He called the spinal cord injury unit at Vancouver General Hospital for advice. One of the spine surgeons answered the call and gave clear instructions: start a corticosteroid protocol, then airlift Frankie to the spinal cord unit immediately.

As the orthopaedic resident on the spine service, I had an opportunity to chat with Dr. Fredrickson a short time later. He was grateful to be able to send Frankie for this highly specialized care and appreciated the specifics of the corticosteroid protocol—a treatment approach with which he was not familiar.

An hour after arriving at the emergency room in Prince George and two hours after his injury, Frankie was in an ambulance heading to the airport. He arrived at Vancouver General Hospital's spinal cord ICU three hours later—a terrified young man still not fully comprehending what had happened to him. The specialized spine nurses and I met him, and got him admitted to the unit. His vital signs were checked, his blood was drawn, and a detailed exam was performed. All the while, we explained what we were doing, answered his questions, and comforted him as best we could. His exam did show complete paralysis, except for retained sensation on his rectal exam—a positive sign.

The on-call spine surgeon arrived. He was one of three spine surgeons who ran the spinal cord injury unit. He had advanced training in spine surgery, and his entire clinical and research practice was devoted to problems related to the spine. He helped me apply traction tongs by anesthetizing the area of the skull just above the ears and then drilling into the skull—just deep enough to place a traction pin, so steady traction could be applied to reduce the dislocated cervical vertebrae.

With gradually increasing traction, the dislocation was reduced and confirmed with x-rays. Subsequently, an MRI was obtained, and a day later Frankie underwent surgery to fuse the unstable cervical spine. For the first four days, he was monitored continuously in the spinal cord ICU. When he had stabilized, he was transferred to the rehabilitation ward, where highly specialized physical therapists worked with him intensely during the following weeks.

I wish I could tell you Frankie regained all of his muscle function and walked normally again, but he did not. However, he did regain some movement in his upper extremity and was able to function independently in a wheelchair. His dedication to the recovery process, aided by the committed and highly-skilled staff at the spinal cord unit, allowed him to optimize the results of this devastating injury.

Frankie was one of three patients with a major spine injury admitted to the spinal cord unit that week. Treating patients with these types of catastrophic injuries was routine for those working in the spinal cord injury unit. I assumed every large trauma hospital had a similar spinal cord injury unit. However, as I spent time training and working at other major orthopaedic centres in North America, I realized I was wrong. The volume of patients, the concentrated expertise, and the coordination among those treating these patients at Vancouver General Hospital's spinal cord injury unit was exceptional. Only a few places in North America had this experience.

In the ensuing years, as they published research on their experiences with various treatment approaches, those leading the spinal cord injury unit became recognized as world leaders. The unit epitomized what I and many others think the Canadian healthcare system should be: highly-trained healthcare experts working in a coordinated manner to render consistently excellent care to a high volume of patients with a specific type of clinical problem. Additionally, patients do not bear any out-of-pocket costs, and there is the opportunity to perform groundbreaking clinical research. The potential for true clinical excellence within the Canadian healthcare system is astonishing.

"Canada has an excellent healthcare system!" This statement used to be heard a lot. Many Canadians still believe it to be true. I believed it myself before my return to Canada in 2010. However, those who may still believe this statement have an idealized view of the present day healthcare system. Often they are citizens without any meaningful interaction with the system, or patients who have been fortunate enough to encounter a pocket of excellence, such as that delivered by the spinal cord injury unit. However, more and more evidence suggests otherwise. This chapter looks at the results of care within the Canadian system and reviews the various factors that prevent the system from consistently delivering high-quality care.

Canadians are slowly waking up to the realization that their healthcare system is far from perfect, that patients often fail to get good care, and that taxpayers are not getting good value for their tax dollars. The Commonwealth Fund is a nonpartisan, private foundation based in the United States, whose goal is to promote a high-performing healthcare system that achieves better access, improved quality, and greater efficiency.[36] As mentioned earlier, in 2010, they rated seven industrialized health systems (Canada, The United States, New Zealand,

---

[36] The Commonwealth Fund: The Funds Mission, Goals, and Strategy. 2012 p 2 2012 http://www.commonwealthfund.org/~/media/Files/Annual%20 Report/2013/Mission_goals_2012.pdf

Australia, Germany, The Netherlands, and the United Kingdom).[37] Despite being the second most expensive system among the seven, Canada ranked last in quality. They defined quality as a combination of safe care, effective care, coordinated care, and patient-centred care. In the 2014 Commonwealth Report, four additional nations were added (Norway, Sweden, France, and Switzerland). Canada was rated second to last overall and 9th out of 11 in the Quality subcategory—still last among the seven nations of the 2010 report (Table 1).[38]

It may not be possible for a single report to fully encapsulate an entire healthcare system's performance. However, despite some arenas of excellence, Canada's healthcare system is not well respected internationally—especially when compared with substantially less expensive systems that offer superior performance in countries like the United Kingdom, Australia, and Sweden.

---

[37] Mirror, Mirror on the Wall: How the Performance of the US Health Care System Compares Internationally 2010 Update. The Commonwealth Fund. Eds: Karen Davis, Cathy Schoen, and Kristof Stremikis. June 2010

[38] The Commonwealth Fund: Mirror, Mirror on the Wall: How the Performance of the US Health System Compares Internationally. Eds: Karen Davis, Kristof Stremikis, David Squires, Cathy Schoen. June 2014. P. 7

Table 1: Commonwealth Fund: Overall Ranking of Healthcare Systems

EXHIBIT ES-1. OVERALL RANKING

COUNTRY RANKINGS
- Top 2*
- Middle
- Bottom 2*

	AUS	CAN	FRA	GER	NETH	NZ	NOR	SWE	SWIZ	UK	US
OVERALL RANKING (2013)	4	10	9	5	5	7	7	3	2	1	11
Quality Care	2	9	8	7	5	4	11	10	3	1	5
Effective Care	4	7	9	6	5	2	11	10	8	1	3
Safe Care	3	10	2	6	7	9	11	5	4	1	7
Coordinated Care	4	8	9	10	5	2	7	11	3	1	6
Patient-Centered Care	5	8	10	7	3	6	11	9	2	1	4
Access	8	9	11	2	4	7	6	4	2	1	9
Cost-Related Problem	9	5	10	4	8	6	3	1	7	1	11
Timeliness of Care	6	11	10	4	2	7	8	9	1	3	5
Efficiency	4	10	8	9	7	3	4	2	6	1	11
Equity	5	9	7	4	8	10	6	1	2	2	11
Healthy Lives	4	8	1	7	5	9	6	2	3	10	11
Health Expenditures/Capita, 2011**	$3,800	$4,522	$4,118	$4,495	$5,099	$3,182	$5,669	$3,925	$5,643	$3,405	$8,508

Notes: * Includes ties. ** Expenditures shown in $US PPP (purchasing power parity); Australian $ data are from 2010.
Source: Calculated by The Commonwealth Fund based on 2011 International Health Policy Survey; 2012 International Health Policy Survey of Sicker Adults; 2013 International Health Policy Survey of Primary Care Physicians; 2013 International Health Policy Survey; Commonwealth Fund National Scorecard 2011; World Health Organization; and Organization for Economic Cooperation and Development, OECD Health Data, 2013 (Paris: OECD, Nov. 2013).

Mediocre Care: Blame the System, Not the Individual

Mediocre medical care within the Canadian healthcare system is the product of many recurring themes. Almost all of these problems can be traced, directly or indirectly, back to the structure of the healthcare system itself. The system has been organized so that care is delivered by siloed groups of doctors, nurses, physical therapists, and administrators. This leads to fragmented, disconnected care—when an integrated, team-based approach is needed.

Unfortunately, the coordinated, consistent clinical excellence that I witnessed in the Vancouver General Hospital's spinal cord injury unit in 1992 was the exception, not the norm. Why? Perhaps because the spinal cord injury unit was relatively new when I worked there; it is almost always easier to build something from scratch than to undo ingrained cultural norms. Perhaps it was the strong dynamic leader of the unit, who created a culture of excellence by force of will and personality. It may have been the nature of the injuries that attract passionate, caring nurses, physiotherapists, and doctors who commit to working together. Maybe it had not yet had time to be swallowed up by the bureaucratic behemoth that accompanies most aspects of the healthcare system.

The success I witnessed there is cause for optimism. It is possible to do very good things within the Canadian healthcare system. Unfortunately, more and more of these types of successes occur in spite of, not because of, the overlying administrative and organizational structure.

So what are the problems inherent in the Canadian healthcare system? There is a variety of recurring system issues that undermine the delivery of quality healthcare. They include:

1. Fragmented care delivery that fails to focus on the patient's overall episode of care.
2. Administrators who make important decisions that directly affect patient care, despite being disconnected from the patient care arena.
3. A near absence of valid and useful outcome metrics which prevents the true results of care from being observed, and when outcomes are reviewed, the results are often not acted upon.

4. Compensation via the fee-for-service model often rewards mediocre care and discourages high-quality care.
5. Poor communication between healthcare providers is the norm, simply because of the way care delivery is organized.
6. A lack of coordination of care, especially between primary care physicians and specialists.
7. A lack of competition and accountability among healthcare providers for patients and jobs ensures that poorly-performing physicians and other healthcare providers retain their positions year after year.

All of these reasons are a direct or indirect product of the Canadian healthcare system itself. The way the system has been organized makes it highly likely that care will continue to be delivered in this manner. This is not about individual doctors, nurses, and administrators functioning poorly, but rather, it is a predictable consequence of the organizational structure. "Each system is perfectly designed to get the results that it does,"[39] and the Canadian healthcare system that I witnessed bears this out. The end result is care that is consistently mediocre—and at times downright atrocious.

1. Wound Infections: fragmented organization of care leads to poor results

After practicing in Canada for about six months, I came to the realization that my post-surgical infection rate had increased significantly. Wound infections in my previous practice in San Francisco had been uncommon—about 1% (2 to 3 patients per year). Now I noted that once or even twice a month, I was seeing a wound infection. Fortunately, most were resolved with antibiotics in time, but nevertheless, this finding was very disconcerting to me.

During the same time, I noted disturbing behaviour patterns within the operating room. Among the OR nurses, there was virtually no

---

[39] This quote has been variously attributed to a variety of individuals, including Institute of Heath Improvement CEO Donald Berwick, quality guru Edwards Deming, and even erroneously, Albert Einstein. It is believed to have originated with Dr. Paul Batalden. (http://www.psqh.com/julaug08/editor.html)

standardization in their approach to sterile technique. A few nurses were outstanding, but most were mediocre with regular violations of sterile technique, while some nurses were downright abysmal—regularly demonstrating a disregard for commonly accepted sterile technique practices. It was not that nurses and other operating room staff were consciously violating sterile technique, but rather, they did not seem to understand the concept and principles.

I noted other troubling behaviours. Coffee was drunk inside the operating rooms. Many of the anesthesiologists would allow their masks to fall loosely around their necks or have their noses exposed. Lab coats used to cover surgical scrubs outside of the operating area were not being removed in the operating areas. Traffic in and out of each operating room was considerable; traffic is known to stir up microscopic particles that carry bacteria every time the door opens.[40] Finally, operating room employees, doctors, nurses, and cleaners regularly went outside—down the street for coffee or across the street to the dog park—in their scrubs and shoes and then returned to the operating room without changing.

When confronted with these types of breaks in accepted sterile technique, my approach was to talk with each person in question individually. When I did this, I occasionally encountered resistance, but in most instances, the individual involved agreed to change their behaviour and did during that day. However, these types of behaviours quickly reverted back to an unacceptable baseline. The culture of the operating room was that of a laissez-faire approach to sterile technique; that was *just the way things were done*. Making any sort of meaningful change without changing the existing organizational structure was simply not going to happen.

Why were commonly accepted sterile techniques ignored in a widespread fashion? The answer seemed clear. In large part, these behaviours were due to the siloed approach to how care delivery was organized. Most nurses, anesthesiologists, and cleaners are completely

---

[40]   Rush of human traffic in Canadian operating rooms could expose patients to 'disastrous' bacterial infections. Sharon Kirkey, The National Post, September 22nd 2015. http://news.nationalpost.com/health/rush-of-human-traffic-in-canadian-operating-rooms-could-expose-patients-to-disastrous-bacterial-infections (accessed November 28th 2015)

divorced from the end results of the surgeries that they were helping to perform in the operating room. Nurses were beholden to the department of operating room nursing, anesthesiologists were beholden to the department of anesthesia, and the cleaning staff responded to their manager.

No one except the surgeon was oriented around the episode of care—the ultimate result that the patient would receive. The surgeon was the only individual who would follow the patient from the start of their surgical treatment through to the finish. The surgeon was usually the only healthcare provider who observed how the patient ultimately fared.

Without a more team-based approach that would allow for easy feedback on the ultimate results of each patient's care, there was no impetus for nurses, anesthesiologists, and others to change their actions. Had they been organized as a team, all oriented to the ultimate results of the patient's experience, things would have been very different. It would have been much easier to explain why strict adherence to sterile technique was critical, to entertain any concerns or difficulties they had in instituting these changes, and to create a culture where everyone respected the need for sterile technique—because they would directly see the results of poor sterile technique.

The logical step would be to move to a team-based approach, also known as a *service line* approach, to care. This movement has been occurring throughout the world, but has been largely absent in Canada. However, breaking down existing departments and reorienting individuals to a different team requires a whole new power structure. Those losing power will fight this move with great force. Yet it is this type of entrenched structure that is largely responsible for the poor, fragmented, and expensive care that is delivered within the Canadian healthcare system.

2. The Twilight Zone: when administrators are disconnected from care delivery

"No! No! I can't take the pain anymore! Please don't let them do this to me!" An 87-year-old woman screamed this at me when I told her that her hip fracture surgery would be delayed. The previous day, Mrs. G had been walking home from her neighborhood coffee shop after visiting with her friends when she tripped and broke her hip—a problem that affects three to five patients per week at my hospital. She had been medically cleared for surgery and had been lying in bed since her arrival, unable to move. The slightest movement of her right leg sent waves of pain radiating from her hip.

It was 2:10 p.m., and I had just finished my orthopaedic trauma slate. My assigned operating room *trauma time* ended at 3:30 p.m. However, Betty, the operating room charge nurse, would not allow Mrs. G's surgery to proceed because her surgery likely would run past 3:30 p.m. Despite a very pleasant demeanor, Betty was often referred to as the *clipboard dictator* because she worked ruthlessly to ensure that none of the operating rooms went over the allotted time.

However, Mrs. G's hip fracture was the very first case on the *emergency add-on list*—the list of emergency cases to be performed outside of the elective operating room time. Despite being at the head of the line, her 90-minute surgery had to wait—and wait—until 7:30 or 8:00 p.m. Mrs. G had become trapped in the *twilight zone*—a three- to five-hour period each afternoon and evening during which NO emergency cases are performed.

In the intervening five hours, Mrs. G was bumped by an emergent appendectomy—an almost inevitable occurrence. It would be 10:00p.m. before the OR staff called for the case and 10:30 p.m. before we could start operating. However, starting that late would have violated one of the hospital's well-founded policies of performing only life- or limb-threatening surgery after 11 p.m.[41] So Mrs. G, who had been lying in bed with her broken hip and fasting all day, had her surgery postponed until the next day.

The story of Mrs. G and the twilight zone illustrates the negative effect on patient care due to administrators who are disconnected from the healthcare playing field organizing the delivery of care—a ubiquitous problem within the Canadian healthcare system. In the example of the twilight zone, coordination and scheduling of the operating rooms was performed by administrators who were not regularly present in the surgical area. Decisions are made that, to the uninitiated, may look good on paper (e.g., demanding that all surgeries finish by 3:30p.m.,

---

41 Culinane, M., et al. "Who Operates When (WOW II)". London: National Confidential Enquiry into Perioperative Deaths (NCEPOD), 2003. **PDF** File. Web.

believing that all nursing and anesthesia staff are interchangeable), but they lead to predictably poor results in the actual delivery of care. In the case of the twilight zone, a failure of administrators understanding how good care needs to be delivered led to poor organization—more specifically the means by which emergency surgeries get performed in a timely manner.

Some variation of the twilight-zone scenario happened at least two or three times per week at my hospital. Emergency surgical patients pay a big price for these twilight-zone delays. Hip-fracture patients, usually elderly individuals, often spend an additional day immobilized in bed due to such delays, significantly increasing the chance that they will develop a complication such as pneumonia or a urinary tract infection.[42,43] All the while, they receive increased amounts of pain medication that clouds their senses and often produces a delirium that precludes early rehab.

In cases of appendicitis and other acute emergencies, delays mean a greater chance that the appendix will rupture or that other such complications will occur.[44] It also means the surgeon will likely be operating in the middle of the night, which greatly affects surgical quality.[45] The existence of the twilight zone increases complications and mortality.

Prior to returning to Canada, I had never heard of an operating room *twilight zone*. All of the hospitals at which I had previously worked

[42]   Novack V, Jotkowitz A, Etzion O, Porath A. Does delay in surgery after hip fracture lead to worse outcomes? A multicenter survey. *International Journal for Quality in Health Care*. DOI: http://dx.doi.org/10.1093/intqhc/mzm003 170-176 First published online: 19 February 2007

[43]   Lefaivre KA, Macadam SA, Davidson DJ, Gandhi R, Chan H, Broekhuyse HM. Length of stay, mortality, morbidity and delay to surgery in hip fractures. *J Bone Joint Surg Br.* 2009 Jul;91(7):922-7. doi: 10.1302/0301-620X.91B7.22446.

[44]   Access to Emergency Operative Care: A Comparative Study Between the Canadian and American Healthcare systems. CJ Brown, SR Finlayson, M C Taylor, (for the members of the Evidence-based Reviews in Surgery Group). Canadian Journal of Surgery Vol 54, No. 6, December 2011 pp. 403-406.

[45]   Ricci, W.M., K. Coupe, R.K. Leighton, et. al. "Is after hours surgery associated with adverse outcomes?" *The American Academy of Orthopaedic Surgeons 72nd Annual Meeting.* Washington, D.C. 23-27 Feb.2005.

addressed this issue in a similar manner—with a potential solution that would work in Canada. They designated a room for emergency surgeries, and when the daytime trauma list was finished, the team in this room immediately began the first case on the *emergency add-on list*. There was a nursing team assigned to this emergency operating room, and the department of anesthesia assigned first, second, and third "day-call" anesthetists to ensure there was always a dedicated anesthesiologist available.[46] Before starting at the hospital in question, I assumed erroneously that all hospitals handled their emergency cases in this logical, coordinated manner.

Addressing this problem does not require any new resources. It just requires that administrative decisions be made by individuals who understand the issues—specifically people who actually take care of patients. Fostering a patient-centred approach to healthcare administration is a central reason why many highly successful health systems, including the Cleveland Clinic, the Mayo Clinic, and the Kaiser Health system, have aggressively promoted clinician leadership.[47,48,49] The operating room *twilight zone* at my hospital has been tolerated for years and tacitly been deemed acceptable. Individual physicians and nurses quickly learn that they are unable to enact meaningful change, so they eventually stop trying. Meanwhile, the administrators who are

---

[46] The anesthetic day-call schedule designates which anesthesiologists will stay late on any given day. As an example, the third day-call anesthetist would not go home until there were only two ORs running, etc.

[47] http://my.clevelandclinic.org/about-cleveland-clinic/overview/leadership

[48] V F Trastek, N W Hamilton, E E Niles, Leadership Models in Health Care—A Case for Servant Leadership. Mayo Clinic Proceedings, Vol 89(3), p 374–381, March 2014

[49] "Working in cooperation with health plan and facility managers, (Kaiser) Permanente physicians take responsibility for clinical care, quality improvement, resource management, and the design and operation of the care delivery system in each region."
D McCarthy, K Mueller, J Wrenn. Kaiser Permanente: Bridging the Quality Divide with Integrated Practice, Group Accountability, and Health Information Technology. Case Study Organized Health Care delivery System. The Commonwealth Fund, p. 3, June 2009.

actually in charge rarely see the direct effects of the system they are leading, and are unable or unwilling to make the needed changes.

This twilight zone example highlights a quality-of-care problem within the operating rooms, caused by the manner in which the system was managed. However, poor management decisions from well-intentioned but disconnected administrators were not confined to the operating rooms at my institution. Rather, administrative disconnect was a recurring theme throughout the system I observed. Furthermore, this was only one of many system issues that regularly undermined the quality of care that the system delivered.

3. Urinary Tract Infections and Catheter Use: outcome metrics to the rescue

The exception proves the rule. Surgeons and nurses at my hospital all knew that some patients developed urinary tract infections (UTIs) due to the inappropriate use of Foley catheters. A Foley or urinary catheter is a tube that is placed into the bladder so patients do not need to urinate. This can be helpful following surgery, when it may not be possible for patients to mobilize to the bathroom, or when very ill patients need their urinary output measured accurately. However, if the urinary catheter is placed incorrectly, if sterile technique is not used, or if it is left in place too long, the result was an infection of the bladder—a UTI. Treating the UTI required removing or replacing the catheter, starting antibiotics, and often prolonging the patient's hospital stays. In some older patients the infection would lead to sepsis and it was necessary to urgently transfer them to the ICU for closer monitoring and more aggressive treatment. Usually they survived, returning to the ward a few days later to recover—but some never returned. The percentage of patients with catheter-related UTIs did not seem high, but uncommon things happen commonly when thousands of patients are treated.

Physicians and nurses at the hospital had in the past attempted to improve the way that Foley catheters were used. Policy papers were developed outlining the correct way to insert and manage Foley catheter, and *in-service* teaching sessions to educate the nurses were held. The staff was receptive and listened intently, but these interventions made no meaningful long-term difference in how catheters were used. One of my colleagues who was involved in these education efforts bluntly stated, "We might as well have been talking to an empty room for all the good it did." The hospital had an established culture; things were just done a certain way. One policy paper or a series of *in-service* teaching sessions was not going to change this culture. But what could?

A year after I arrived at our hospital, we joined The North American Surgical Quality Improvement Program (NSQIP). NSQIP was founded in 1994 by the United States Veterans Administration Hospital system. It subsequently became affiliated with the American College of Surgeons, who now oversee this program. As of 2015, NSQIP has over 640 participating hospitals and surgical centres, including 43 in Canada.

The NSQIP program worked by randomly selecting surgical patients, then measuring preoperative, intra-operative, and 30-day postoperative data. It thereby provided "fair, in-depth and insightful analysis, helping surgeons and hospitals better understand their quality of care compared to similar hospitals with similar patients."[50] Complications such as heart attacks, blood clots, UTIs, wound-healing problems, and hospital readmission were measured and compared to other equivalent hospitals throughout North America. This provided an accurate, standardized assessment of surgical performance, albeit for a limited number of parameters, compared to similar hospitals.

Among the outliers in the first set of NSQIP results for our hospital were UTIs. They were almost three times the national average (4.7% vs. 1.62%), and this was directly attributable to improper catheter use. Faced with inescapable, hard data that demanded action, nurses, doctors, and administrators mobilized. Another educational program was created to improve the way that catheters were used in surgical cases. In this instance, the impetus for change highlighted by the outcome metrics was perceived as very real. The intervention was widely accepted, and relatively quickly, the urinary tract infection rate began to decline. Hard, accurate outcome metrics had done what previous teaching sessions, policy papers, and respected clinical leaders had failed to achieve—fundamentally change the culture.

---

[50]   http://site.acsnsqip.org/about/

Unfortunately, NSQIP only measures a relatively small number of complications. It does not measure outcomes that are surgery-specific, and it is not being used in most hospitals in Canada. NSQIP's impact is still limited. However, it does provide opportunities in certain areas (i.e., to see how one hospital is performing relative to other hospitals), and this knowledge can be a powerful driver of change.

NSQIP data was collected independently and prospectively, and therefore tended to be fairly accurate. This was not the case with most healthcare data that was collected. In June 2012, the British Columbia Ministry of Health's official surgical waitlist identified that I had 10 patients waiting for elective foot and ankle surgery.[51] The reality was that in preparation for my departure, I had completed my last elective surgery two months earlier. The figures for my other orthopaedic colleagues—who were still practicing—were similarly inaccurate.

Accurate, transparent outcome metrics are a cornerstone of modern medicine.[52] Unfortunately, in the Canadian medical system that I observed, there were many metrics that were measured, but it seemed that most were either irrelevant or inaccurate. The BC Surgical waitlist was one of many examples I encountered. The end result was a lack of impetus for change. In most instances, the system perpetuates itself.

For administrators, physicians, and other healthcare employees, it is often bad news to see hard, accurate outcome data. This type of data allows direct comparisons to other institutions. Faced with irrefutable data that shows your institution has a higher complication rate, lower patient satisfaction scores, longer lengths of stay, or more monetary spending than an equivalent hospital, difficult choices and significant changes must be made. It is much easier for administrators within the system to not have this information—and therefore not be subject to scrutiny and the need for major upheaval. Yet it is exactly this hard, accurate outcome data that is needed in order to move the healthcare system forward.

---

[51]   https://swt.hlth.gov.bc.ca/faces/Home.xhtml# (Accessed December 12th, 2015)

[52]   N Henke, T Kelsey, H Whately. Transparency — the most powerful driver of health care improvement? *Health International* is published by McKinsey's Health Systems and Services Practice. Copyright © 2011. McKinsey & Company.

4. *Piecemeal Medicine: the perils of fee-for-service compensation*

"Hopefully your symptoms will settle down, but if they don't, we will have to chat about that during another visit," Dr. Smith said in a friendly voice on his way out the door. My friend Norman liked his primary care physician. Dr. Smith seemed smart and approachable. They had just had a short but productive discussion on the management of Norman's high blood pressure.

However, as Norman changed the topic to his nagging lower back pain, Dr. Smith ended the discussion before it could begin. *One problem per visit* was the unwritten rule at Dr. Smith's office. Aided by his highly-organized assistant Mary, Dr. Smith ran his office on time, and Norman liked this efficiency. However, Norman had become increasingly frustrated by the short visits, the inability to discuss multiple problems, and the relatively reactive treatments he received—usually either a pill or referral.

When Norman's pain failed to resolve, he returned to see Dr. Smith a few weeks later. The doctor asked a few questions and performed a basic physical exam. He recommended some anti-inflammatory medication, avoiding excessive sitting, and some gentle exercise. He also made a referral to an orthopaedic surgeon, as he had concerns that Norman's symptoms may be the result of a bulging disc.

After a two-month wait during which time Norman's symptoms had improved somewhat, he visited an orthopaedic surgeon who ordered a computed tomography (CT) scan of Norman's lower back. This was performed a few weeks later and was negative for a herniated disc. However, there was an unrelated finding. Norman's CT scan identified a somewhat unusual-looking cyst on his right kidney. The report described it as "benign-looking" and recommended "further follow-up."

Norman returned to Dr. Smith to discuss the CT scan findings. Dr. Smith assured him that the cyst was "probably not malignant." To be safe, he referred him for an assessment by a urologist. Norman took the earliest appointment available for the urologist, which was five weeks later. However, two days before the scheduled appointment, the urologist's office phoned and said they would need to reschedule. Norman had to wait another four weeks.

He grew increasingly anxious fearing that this growth on his kidney may be cancerous. He made another appointment with Dr. Smith to discuss the situation. Dr. Smith was kind but firm. The urologist would manage the kidney issue, just as the orthopaedic surgeon was handling his lower back problem. He encouraged Norman to call the urologist's office and see if there were any cancellations, but other than that, he did not have any suggestions.

"Why does Dr. Smith not get more involved in my care?" Norman asked me. "Isn't that what primary care doctors are supposed to do?" I sympathized with Norman's concerns. However, I pointed out that Dr. Smith was behaving exactly how one would have predicted, given how he was compensated.

In the fee-for-service system, physicians like Dr. Smith get paid for each individual interaction with the patient. They do not get paid for the overall coordination of care. He receives $30.15 for each patient he sees.[53] With rent to pay on his office, his assistant Mary's salary, and the other expenses of running a practice, Dr. Smith needs to see a patient every 8-10 minutes in order to make what he would consider a reasonable income for a physician.[54] That is the nature of the existing fee-for-service system. As much as Dr. Smith or other physicians might like to run their practices differently, they are locked into this model, given how they are compensated. This is a source of frustration for many physicians, who went to medical school with the goal of providing the type of care Norman expected.

There are three ways a fee-for-service compensation system adversely affects the quality of healthcare that the Canadian healthcare system delivers. First, it rewards and thereby encourages poor care. In a system where there is a high demand for physician services, the faster the patient is seen (and the less attention to detail the physician pays in examining and treating the patient), the more money the physician

---

[53] In-office visit fee for a general practitioner in British Columbia seeing a patient between the ages of 2-49 for a specific complaint. (http://www.health.gov.bc.ca/msp/infoprac/physbilling/payschedule/pdf/7-general-practice.pdf)

[54] Family physicians average income in Canada ranges from $50,483 - $252,006. http://www.healthcare-salaries.com/physicians/primary-care-physician-salary

will earn. Second, as in the case with Dr. Smith, paying for each visit encourages isolated interactions with the physician—and a referral to a specialist at the earliest sign of problems, rather than a more holistic approach that focuses on the entire episode of care. Finally, it precludes meaningful innovation in care delivery. For example, a coordinated, practical, team-based approach that emphasizes allied healthcare professionals working in synch with physicians cannot be introduced in a system with a fee-for-service funding model.

5. Retinal Detachment: a failure in communication

One of my friends is a robust, 73-year-old man named Bob who looks and acts 20 years younger. He works out regularly and still practices full-time as a highly-trained professional. One day, he noticed "floaters and stars" in his right eye. He also noted that one part of his vision was blurry. Naturally, he was alarmed and immediately sought help from his primary care physician. He managed to obtain an appointment that day. Dr. Johnson, his physician, examined him and was also concerned.

The doctor made an emergency referral to an ophthalmologist that he commonly used. He completed the referral form, marked it as urgent, and had his assistant fax it over to the ophthalmologist's office. Dr. Johnson must have felt his job was done: identify an urgent problem, send it in the right direction, and move on with a busy day.

Unfortunately, the ophthalmologist's office had a new administrative assistant, and the ophthalmologist was heading off on vacation for a week. The end result was that the ophthalmologist in question did not see this referral until 10 days later. Upon finally seeing the referral, the ophthalmologist scheduled Bob for an urgent visit. A retinal detachment was diagnosed, and he was operated on shortly thereafter. Fortunately, he made a nearly full recovery, but on a regular basis, many patients are not so fortunate.

Communication, or the lack thereof, is a major issue within all healthcare systems. In most industries, there are checks and balances to ensure that critical information gets were it needs to go and is acted upon. This simply does not happen consistently in the fragmented Canadian healthcare system. Poor communication, in all its various forms, seems ubiquitous. Patients like Bob, with life-altering or life-threatening medical conditions, regularly slip through the cracks: lab tests are not checked, and important results are missed. Inadequate handoffs of patients—from physician to physician within hospitals—seem to be the norm. Basic administrative data, such as who is waiting for surgery, is not communicated regularly, with resulting great expense and delays in care.

What is so exasperating about witnessing persistent, dysfunctional communication is not only that it happens so regularly. It is also that in theory, the centralized, provincial oversight of the medical system should allow for the creation of integrated programs that ensure that patient-related communications between primary care physicians, specialists, and other healthcare providers occurs in a seamless manner. However, as will be discussed in greater detail in Chapter 5, the *Canadian healthcare system* is not actually a system; rather, it is primarily a means for the government to fund various elements of healthcare. By continuing with the existing funding model and system organization that promotes fragmentation and non-standardized care, this type of miscommunication is almost guaranteed.

6. *The Referral Wall: a lack of coordination between primary care and specialists*

Shortly after I started my position as head of the department of orthopaedics, I met with one of the leaders of the family medicine department. He expressed his frustrations to me regarding obtaining specialist consultations from my surgical colleagues. I asked him what he meant. He told me, "We cannot get our patients seen in a timely manner. It is so frustrating." At this meeting, I did not fully understand what he was saying. I soon came to see his concerns firsthand.

When a family physician sees a patient that he or she believes needs a specialist consultation, a referral is placed. The family physician needs to decide which specialist they would recommend for their patient to visit.

Yet the primary care physician and their patient will not have all the information needed to make an informed decision. They do not know the wait time to see the specialist (Wait Time #1), or even whether that individual is actually interested in seeing new patients. If it is a potential surgical case, they do not know how long each specialist's waitlist for surgery might be after seeing the surgeon (Wait Time #2). There is no central repository to coordinate specialist referrals. Once the referral has been submitted, the family physician often loses oversight of that patient, with respect to the clinical problem in question. The patient is often left to confront the "referral wall" on their own.

I quickly came to see that the specialists on the other end of this equation often had very different agendas. Some specialists did not want to see patients in consultation, or they cherry-picked cases that they would find interesting or would likely lead to surgery. Others only wanted to see enough to keep their surgical waitlist up to a reasonable level. This created artificially long versions of *Wait Time #1* that served to drive people to get their care in private clinics—where they would charge \$400-\$700 to see a patient, instead of the provincial healthcare fee of approximately \$100.[55] Still other specialists would see patients relatively quickly and then create a very long surgical *Wait Time #2*, hoping to drive patients to their private surgical practice.

The referral process was completely disorganized. No one in the system was coordinating it. Individual physicians were simply allowed to do what was in their best interests. Doctors were, after all, technically private business owners. There was no individual or group within the healthcare system whose primary job was to represent and advocate for the needs of specific patient groups. The "referral wall"—and the associated difficulty with accessing care—was just another example of how the system, or lack thereof, promoted dysfunctional, expensive care.

7. The Worst Orthopaedic Surgeon in British Columbia: a lack of competition and accountability among healthcare providers

Who is the worst orthopaedic surgeon in the province of British Columbia? This is an entirely subjective question that likely could never be answered, but what if the question was, "Who do orthopaedic surgeons

---

[55]   Private practice outside of the provincial healthcare systems is technically illegal under the Canada Health Act for physicians who are practicing within the public system. However, some physicians find ways to see patients who pay privately for expedited appointments or surgeries.

in BC think is the worst orthopaedic surgeon in the province?" Ask this question in public, and you will invariably get diplomatic responses like, "All of my colleagues are highly trained," or, "No comment!" Ask this question to an orthopaedic surgeon in private, and one name will come up time and time again: an individual whose poor judgment, lack of attention to detail, and long history of malpractice litigation is well known.

Despite this record of perceived incompetence, this individual's medical staff privileges are fully secure. This, combined with an oversupply of patients relative to the existing physician services, means there will always be work for this surgeon. Like many other physicians, this individual simply does not have to compete for their jobs. In general, nothing short of a felony conviction will prevent established physicians from retaining their hospital privileges once they have secured a full-time hospital appointment.

Furthermore, hospitals do not open up spots for new physicians based on patient demand or the desire to outcompete a low-performing physician. Rather, they are usually based on whether there is adequate funding to support the new physician. The result is a de facto monopoly position for many physicians within the Canadian healthcare system.

Contrast this with the 1 out of 6 new orthopaedic surgeon graduates who cannot find a permanent job.[56] These young surgeons have just spent ten years or more undergoing rigorous training (four years in medical school, five years in a surgical residency, and one or more years in subspecialty fellowship training). They are some of Canada's most dynamic and accomplished young adults, yet many cannot find a job. Some go from one locum (substituting for an orthopaedic surgeon who is away) to another, or they may cover emergency on-call shifts at a hospital for a short period. Others move to the United States, where their expertise is welcomed with open arms.

There is no way of knowing whether the "worst orthopaedic surgeon" is deserving of this reputation. However, if quality is a central

---

[56]   Are Canadian medical schools graduating the doctors of yesterday? This study finds 1 in 6 specialists can't find work: Canadian Press and National Post Staff | October 10, 2013. http://news.nationalpost.com/news/doctor-shortages-a-myth-nearly-one-in-six-new-medical-specialists-cant-find-work-report-suggests (accessed April 18, 2015)

goal of the healthcare system, this physician, and all physicians, should be subject to some competition as a prerequisite for retaining their jobs. If competition were allowed, this surgeon, and many other physicians, would be steadily supplanted by better-trained, harder-working, and more responsive physicians.

Serious competition among physicians within the existing Canadian healthcare system does not happen to any meaningful extent. In fact, actions by medical staffs, and provincial doctors' groups, specifically discourage this type of competition. This takes many forms, but the end result is that physicians in established positions protect their turf; no doubt, the same can be said for administrators and other healthcare professionals. It is a natural human reaction. However, failure to promote any type of meaningful competition within the healthcare system is a major impediment to ensuring consistently high-quality patient care.

Mediocre Care by Design: Consistently Violating the Principles of Providing Good Healthcare

Each of the examples in this chapter illustrates a failure to adhere to one or more of the principles of providing high-quality, modern healthcare.

- The regular violation of sterile technique in the operating room highlights one of the many problems associated with a siloed approach to care delivery, whereby most healthcare workers do not receive feedback on their performance—with respect to how the patient ultimately fared.
- Mrs. G's delayed hip surgery due to the *twilight zone* illustrates the problems that can occur when administrators try to organize care delivery, despite being disconnected from the delivery process.
- The elevated urinary tract infection rate, due to poor catheter use, demonstrates the difficulty of changing cultures in the absence of accurate outcome metrics.
- Norman's experience with his primary care physician, Dr. Smith, highlights how the fee-for-service compensation system drives care delivery patterns that do not promote quality healthcare.

- The delay in the diagnosis of Bob's retinal detachment illustrates the critical importance of communication within the healthcare system—something that is difficult or impossible in Canada's fragmented system.
- The *referral wall* demonstrates the dysfunction, and resulting difficulty, accessing specialist care that occurs when each practitioner functions in isolation—according to their own best interests, rather than as a part of a coordinated, larger whole.
- Finally, the tale of the *worst orthopaedic surgeon* highlights the distinct lack of competition that presently exists within the system, and thereby fails to weed out underperforming physicians, administrators, and other healthcare providers.

What is striking about all of these issues is that they are directly or indirectly attributable to how the system itself is organized. The system has created these impediments to quality healthcare—either by structuring healthcare delivery in such a way that these types of problems are inevitable, or by creating a perverse incentive system that encourages or, at a minimum, fails to penalize dysfunctional behaviours.

Summary: Chapter 3

Winning hockey games, being consistently successful throughout the regular hockey season, and performing well in the Stanley Cup playoffs is all about team performance. The coach and general manager make countless decisions that are all oriented to producing results. Who should be on the team? Which players should play in specific games? Which players should be benched, traded, or sent to the minor leagues? What is the team's strategy for success? These are just a few of the many questions that need to be answered.

If they are answered correctly, the team will win, and the coach and general manager will be rewarded with new contracts and more money. If the coach and general manager are unsuccessful, they will be fired. They understand the expectations. Failure is not an option.

Consider an *episode of care* such as treating a patient with cancer or providing surgical care (e.g., managing a hip fracture) as akin to a single hockey game. In this instance, treating multiple patients with similar cancers, or multiple patients with hip fractures, is the equivalent of a team's hockey season. By this analogy, the healthcare system can be broken down into a variety of different "teams," each responsible for treating patients with a specific condition or similar conditions throughout their episode of care.

To be successful, all of the *players on the team* must share a common goal: obtaining optimal care for the patient. They must work as a coordinated team and understand the results of their team's care. They must be committed to the team and its goals, but also must understand that they will each be held accountable for their individual responsibilities. Finally, each *team* must have clear leadership. A *coach* is needed to manage each individual episode of care, and a *general manager* is required to oversee all of the care in that area. As in hockey, the coach and general manager need to be able to oversee the entire episode of care, understand how all the component parts fit together, have the ability to alter the team to optimize performance, and be held fully accountable for the team's performance.

However, the standard approach to healthcare delivery in Canada does not resemble anything like a coordinated, team-based approach. Teams are not assembled based on the varied players required to achieve a coordinated healthcare team. Rather, they are grouped by position (centres, wingers, left defense, right defense, goalie, etc.)—each affiliated largely with their own kind, and interacting with the other positions only out of necessity.

Furthermore, very few of the "players" ever know the "final score" (how the patient actually did). Everyone is encouraged to give their best, but except in very rare instances of egregious behaviours, no one is held accountable for their performance. Additionally, there is no head coach to coordinate the team, and if there is a general manager, he or she is likely to be completely disconnected from what is happening—and is not held accountable for performance in any meaningful way. Given this disorganization, it is not surprising and instead expected that the Canadian healthcare system delivers mediocre care. Canadians pay for and deserve a healthcare system that is more than a perennial cellar dweller.

Summary Points: Chapter 3

Canadians are slowly waking up to the realization that their healthcare system is far from perfect, that patients often fail to get good care, and that taxpayers are not getting the value their tax dollars pay for.

Mediocre care within the Canadian healthcare system is the product of many recurring issues. Almost all of these problems can be traced, directly or indirectly, back to the structure of the healthcare system itself. The system has been organized so that care is delivered by siloed groups of doctors, nurses, other healthcare professionals, and administrators. This leads to fragmented, disconnected care—when an integrated, team-based approach is needed.

Recurring system issues that undermine the delivery of quality healthcare in Canada include:

1. Fragmented care delivery that fails to focus on the patient's total episode of care.
2. Administrators who make important decisions that directly affect patient care, despite being disconnected from the patient-care arena.
3. A near absence of valid and useful outcome metrics which prevent the true results of care from being observed, and when outcomes *are* reviewed, the results are often not acted upon.
4. Compensation via a fee-for-service model that rewards mediocre care and discourages high-quality care.
5. Poor communication between healthcare providers is the norm, simply because of the way care delivery is organized.
6. A lack of coordination of care, especially between primary care physicians and specialists.
7. A lack of competition and accountability among healthcare providers for patients and jobs ensures that poorly-performing physicians and other healthcare providers retain their positions year after year.

CHAPTER 4

A Brief History of Medicine

Hockey appears to have originated in Windsor, Nova Scotia. Circa 1800, students from King's College School, Canada's first college, began playing the fast-paced Irish game of hurling on ice.[58] By the early 1890s, hockey clubs were ubiquitous in eastern Canada. One of the most well-known teams was the Rideau Hall Rebels. Playing in Ottawa, the team was made up of parliamentarians and government "aide-de-camps."[59] Team members included William and Arthur Stanley, two sons of Governor General Lord Fredrick Stanley of Preston, the 16th Earl of Derby.

Lord Stanley became so enamoured with the sport he watched his sons play, that in 1893 he purchased a Silver Bowl for $48.57 to be awarded to Canada's top-ranking amateur hockey club.[60] This bowl was originally known as the Dominion Hockey Challenge Cup, but it was soon referred to as the Stanley Cup—now emblematic of hockey supremacy.[61]

One hundred years ago, hockey players looked very different than the players we see flying around the ice today in the National Hockey League (NHL). Early hockey equipment was rudimentary. Goalies began wearing pads, adapted from the pads that wicket keepers wore when playing cricket. Skaters began placing magazines between their shins and their socks, in order to protect their lower legs from being slashed or struck by a puck.

---

57   http://www.birthplaceofhockey.com/origin/overview/
58   http://www.birthplaceofhockey.com/origin/jga-creighton-ottawa/
59   http://www.sportsknowhow.com/hockey/history/hockey-history.shtml
60   http://en.wikipedia.org/wiki/Stanley_Cup

The game was also dramatically different. Players played the entire game with no substitutions. Teams played a rigid, positional style of hockey, with each player concentrating on their own area and responsibility. No forward passes were allowed, which placed an emphasis on the rushing skills of individual players. The players themselves were different—they were often fit by the standards of the day, yet many of them smoked. Year-round, hockey-specific training was unimaginable.

The rules and nature of the game itself also evolved. In 1900, the Halifax Crescents, playing against the Montreal Shamrocks for the Stanley Cup, added fish netting to the metal goal posts—making it easier to clarify that a goal had been scored.[62] The Halifax team lost, but the netting on the goals stayed. In 1913, Frank and Lester Patrick introduced zones in hockey by adding two blue lines, and the rules were changed to allow forward passes within each zone.[63] Hockey quickly became popular throughout the country, and it was not uncommon to have a thousand or more paying spectators, which made it a lucrative endeavour for team owners.

Equipment continued to improve. Newer shin pads were designed. Players began using padded gloves to protect their hands in the early 1900s, and padded hockey pants were added around 1910.[64] Sticks became lighter, and in the 1940s, laminated wood was added to the blade; a final layer of fiberglass was added in the 1960s. Still, none of the players wore helmets, and even goaltenders did not wear masks until Jacques Plante of the Montreal Canadians began wearing one in 1959.

[61]   http://www.thepeoplehistory.com/icehockeyhistory.html

[62]   http://www.thepeoplehistory.com/icehockeyhistory.html

[63]   http://www.stickshack.com/Hockey-Equipment-History.htm

The best hockey players became professionals, playing in the NHL. Stars, such as Howie Morenz in the 1920s and 1930s and Rocket Richard and Gordie Howe in the 1940s and 1950s, helped extend the boundaries of skills and toughness for the players of that era. Players became better skaters, passing improved, and shots became more accurate. By 1967, when the Toronto Maple Leafs won the Stanley Cup, their team bore only a passing resemblance to the teams that had played 50 years earlier.

However, spurred by the influence of Soviet and European styles of hockey, the NHL game underwent a transformation in the 1980 and 1990s. This influence emphasized team play and passing to create scoring chances. Led by the wizardry of players like Wayne Gretzky, teams began to play at a higher level and in a more coordinated way than had ever been seen before.

Today's professional hockey players are noticeably dissimilar from the Toronto Maple Leafs' last Stanley Cup championship team of 1967. They wear lightweight protective equipment, covering almost every area of their body. Everyone wears a helmet, and all of the goalies wear masks and helmets. The players train intensely year-round—not just for fitness, but to hone high-level hockey skills. More fundamentally, they bring team play to a completely different level; every player understands that their job requires them to be part of a larger integrated whole.

Introduction: *An Overview of the History of Modern Medicine*

To envision the medical system of the future, it is critical to understand how the delivery of medical care has evolved. The practice of medicine can be viewed as having three broad eras. The first era, existing prior to 1900, was an era of *magical thinking*. The second era, starting roughly at the turn of the 20ᵗʰ century, could be labeled the *pioneering era*. Finally, the third era began around the year 2000 and can be considered the era of *systematized care delivery*.

The man many consider to be the founding father of modern medicine was a Canadian.[64] Sir William Osler was born in Bond Head, Canada West, in 1849. He spent much of his childhood in Dundas, Ontario. Both his mother and father were very religious, and they had hopes that their son would be a minister. In 1867, Osler entered the ministry and enrolled at Trinity College, located in Weston, Ontario. However, he quickly became fascinated by the emerging field of medical science and began taking medical classes.

In due course, Osler was accepted to the McGill University School of Medicine in Montreal. He graduated with an MDCM degree in 1872, and after some advanced medical training in Europe, Osler returned to McGill as a professor in 1874. While at McGill, he pioneered the use of a journal club—reviewing published articles from the "scientific" literature as a means of teaching students.

Osler left McGill to join the faculty at the University of Pennsylvania in 1884. In 1885, he was one of the seven founding members of the Association of American Physicians, an organization committed to the "advancement of scientific and practical medicine." In 1889, Osler was appointed as Physician-in-Chief of the newly formed Johns Hopkins University School of Medicine and stayed there until 1905, when he took up the post of Regius Chair of Medicine at Oxford.

There are many reasons why Osler is known as the father of modern medicine. He authored *The Principles and Practices of Medicine* in 1892. This comprehensive textbook quickly became one of the primary teaching tools in medicine. It was regularly updated, and it remained

---

[64]   http://en.wikipedia.org/wiki/William Osler

in print until 2001. Osler has been credited with popularizing many foundational, clinical, and educational advances—ideas we take for granted today, but were considered revolutionary in his time. "Listen to your patient; he is telling you the diagnosis," was a common statement he uttered, emphasizing the critical need to "take a history."

Osler was most proud of insisting that medical students see and examine patients, rather than merely listen to lectures. "He who studies medicine without books sails an uncharted sea, but he who studies medicine without patients does not go to sea at all." Seeing and examining real patients as part of the training process to become a physician is obvious in today's world, but it was rare in Olser's day. Medical students in the 1800s typically only received didactic lectures during their medical school training. Osler introduced the clinical clerkship, whereby third- and fourth-year medical students spent time on the hospital wards—learning about clinical medicine and helping to provide patient care. Similarly, he popularized residency training programs, whereby doctors obtain additional training by spending a year or more "in residency" at a hospital after their graduation from medical school.

Osler's ideas were encapsulated in the unique curriculum he oversaw at the newly formed Johns Hopkins School of Medicine. The Hopkins medical program admitted students only after two years of university study, and then provided them with four rigorous years of medical training. The first two years were largely in the classroom: they studied normal anatomy, histology, and physiology in the first year, and then they moved on to didactically review pathological conditions in the second year. The third and fourth years involved innovative medical clerkships in four areas: medicine, surgery, obstetrics, and pathology. Students spent time with patients, under the guidance of teaching physicians. The results were physician graduates who were knowledgeable, experienced, and ready to practice—or ready to enter a residency program to obtain even more detailed training.

Johns Hopkins Medical School trained physicians who were solidly grounded in the science of medicine, who were up-to-date on the latest medical treatments, and who could render treatments that were often effective as a result. Osler's ideas led medicine out of the 19th century, where magical thinking and invoking the as-yet unidentified *placebo effect* were the primary means of treating patients.

At the turn of the 20th century, there were more than 180 "medical schools" in the United States and Canada.[65] They were of widely varying quality. Most medical schools in the 1800s were "for profit" enterprises, often run by a single physician or a small number of physicians who made money from their students' tuitions. Many were only six months in length and required no prerequisite university courses. Prior to 1900, physicians themselves were often not licensed by state or federal authorities, so a diploma was all that was needed to call oneself a "physician." Needless to say, the quality of physicians and medical training was highly variable. Most physicians functioned as businessmen, employing magical thinking or using unusual techniques such as blood letting; others administered pills and potions in order to give patients the impression of competence.

Validation of Osler's ideas about teaching and patient care came in the form of a comprehensive report on medical education, researched and written by American educator Abraham Flexner in 1910. Sensing the wide variation in standards among physicians, the Carnegie Foundation commissioned a report on medical education in 1909. [66] They hired Flexner, a 43-year-old high school teacher and education expert, to write the report. For 16 months, Flexner visited every medical school in the United States and Canada. He asked basic questions, such as: "How long is the program?" "Who makes up the faculty?" And, "Is there an anatomy laboratory?"

The results of his study proved to be transformative. Flexner concluded the vast majority of the 151 medical schools he reviewed were

---

[65] In 1904 there were 160 MD granting institutions (https://en.wikipedia. org/wiki/Flexner_Report). From 1900-1904 an additional 24 medical schools were closed (https://en.wikipedia.org/wiki/ List_of_defunct_medical_schools_in_the_United_States -accessed December 14th 2015)

[66] Medical Education in the United States and Canada: A Report to the Carnegie Foundation for the Advancement of Teaching. Abraham Flexner. 1910 http://archive.carnegiefoundation.org/pdfs/elibrary/ Carnegie_Flexner_Report.pdf

unsatisfactory and should be closed.[67] However, he identified the Johns Hopkins School of Medicine's approach to educating medical students as ideal. He recommended that the Hopkins model of training—two years in the classroom, followed by two years of clinical clerkship rotations in medicine, surgery, obstetrics, and pathology—should become the standard medical curriculum of the future. This report, combined with a movement to license physicians at the state level, led to a revolution in medical education.

By 1920 the number of medical schools in North America had plummeted to 85. More or less, all surviving medical schools provided training based on Osler's Hopkins model: ensuring that physicians were well-grounded in science, skilled in listening to and examining their patients, and up-to-date on the latest medical research.

The Association of American Medical Colleges (AAMC), which had been formed in 1876 to "consider all matters relating to reform in medical college work,"[68] incorporated many of Flexner's proposals in their oversight of the curriculums at these medical schools. The AAMC continues in this role today. This explains why medical schools in the United States and Canada are not considered foreign to each other; they both have the same overseeing body.

Osler had delineated a vision of the 20th century physician: a pioneering individualist. This new kind of physician was grounded in science and committed to the paradigm of taking a history, performing a physical exam, rendering a diagnosis, and then developing a treatment plan; these physicians worked hard. Osler's physician was self-reliant and usually worked alone. Osler was a medical pioneer, who by sheer force of will (and perhaps by the force of his voice), drove people to his way of thinking.

Unlike those physicians practicing magical thinking prior to the 1900s, this 20th century physician had some effective forms of treatment. However, in the early years of the 20th century, before the advent of antibiotics and other treatments, many ailments were still

---

[67] Barzansky, Barbara; Gevitz, Norman (1992). *Beyond Flexner: Medical Education in the Twentieth Century* (1. publ. ed.). New York: Greenwood Press. ISBN 978-0313259845.

[68] https://www.aamc.org/about/history/ Accessed December 13th, 2014

poorly understood or near impossible to treat. Nevertheless, the fact that some treatments were successful—and that there were now fewer physicians who had undergone this more rigorous training—created somewhat of a monopoly for the 20th century physician.

This headstrong, individualistic approach to medicine provided energetic men—the vast majority of 20th century physicians were men— to push the frontier of science-based medicine forward. By the end of the 20th century, spectacular advances had occurred in almost all forms of medical care. However, the paradigm of the hard-working, independent physician made the transition to systematized, team-based care of the 21st century medical system that much more difficult. The 20th century, pioneering physician does not "play well with others."

To more fully understand the issues of incorporating physicians into medical practice today, it is necessary to understand the evolution of the modern physician in more detail.

The Era of Magical Thinking: Pre-1900

Prior to 1900, physicians typically had little formal training and few forms of effective treatment. This is not to imply that no effective treatments existed in the 1800s. However, poor training, a lack of professional standardization, and a very slow diffusion of knowledge and skills meant that most physicians rendered treatment that was of limited effectiveness—and in some instances, made patients worse.

Physicians during this era were competing professionally—with pharmacists, homeopaths, eclectics (botanic doctors), and other healthcare providers—to be recognized as the primary source of healthcare knowledge in the eyes of the public. As the 19th century drew to a close, physicians won this battle, thanks to men like William Osler, who firmly tied medicine (and the physicians who controlled medicine) to science. As science came to be seen in a positive light by the general population, due to developments such as the steam engine and (eventually) flight, those affiliated with science were given more respect. Paul Starr, author of the 1983 Pulitzer Prize-winning book *The Social Transformation of American Medicine*, describes this movement:

"The medical profession has had an especially persuasive claim to authority. Unlike law and the clergy, it enjoys close bonds with modern science, and at least for most of the last century, scientific knowledge has held a privileged status in the hierarchy of belief. ... On this basis, physicians exercise authority over patients, their fellow workers in health care, and even the public at large in matters within, and sometimes outside, their jurisdiction."[69]

A series of revolutionary scientific breakthroughs in medicine and surgery during the 19th century established physicians as the central actors in the developing healthcare system. Physician power was subsequently consolidated and then propagated, leading to a physician-dominated medical system in the 20th century. An exploration of some of these key developments is instructive.

It can be argued that Dr. Edward Jenner started the era of modern medicine in 1796. By inoculating patients with cowpox, he developed and popularized an effective means of preventing smallpox, a devastating illness that came on suddenly, afflicting otherwise healthy individuals and killing 30% of its victims. Those who survived developed hideous scars over their entire body. The condition terrorized entire countries.

Jenner took a simple observation (that milkmaids develop cowpox but never seemed to develop smallpox), developed a hypothesis, and then tested his theory experimentally. Jenner hypothesized that if he could give his patients cowpox, they would not get smallpox. He took pustules from a cowpox skin lesion and spread this into a scratch on the hand of an eight-year-old boy named James Phipps. (Needless to say, ethics panels and institutional review boards were nonexistent at that time.) In a few days, the boy developed redness in his hand, as well as the pustules associated with cowpox. After a few weeks, his symptoms settled. Six weeks later, Jenner exposed the boy to smallpox. The boy developed no symptoms.

---

[69] Paul Starr. *The Social Transformation of American Medicine: The rise of a sovereign profession and the making of a vast industry.* Harper Collins Publishers, 1982. P4-5

Jenner used this technique on many other patients with similar results. In 1797, he wrote up the results of his studies and submitted the paper to the Royal Society. It was rejected—starting a long tradition whereby revolutionary treatments are initially shunned. He subsequently wrote a pamphlet and called this procedure *vaccination*: literally "smallpox of the cow." By 1800, over 100,000 people had been vaccinated in England. This was perhaps the first effective treatment or prevention of a major illness in the history of medicine.

Jenner had ushered in the modern era of medicine. He had found a treatment approach to a devastating illness that actually worked. Yet it would be more than 180 years before smallpox was effectively eradicated.[70]

In the midst of the American Civil War, shortly after delivering the Gettysburg address in November, 1863, President Abraham Lincoln contracted smallpox; so too did his valet William Johnson.[71] They developed high fevers and the classic pustules over their skin. Johnson died; Lincoln lived. The history of the United States—and the results of the Civil War—may have been different had Lincoln perished from smallpox. But why had either of them developed smallpox when an effective prophylactic treatment (vaccination) had existed for over 60 years?

Sadly, a slow diffusion of knowledge and widespread, long-standing delays in implementing effective new treatments were the norm in the 1800s. A lack of standardization in training, a near absence of continuing medical education, and no government mandate of minimum standards of competence often meant that it was decades before new effective treatments were widely available.

The twin medical triumphs of the 19th century were the development of effective anesthesia and Pasteur's germ theory, leading to aseptic technique. Together, these two breakthroughs allowed successful surgery to be performed. In 1800, the need to undergo surgery (for example, the amputation of a gangrenous leg) was rightly considered a terrifying undertaking. Barbers performed surgeries; no self-respecting

---

[70]   http://en.wikipedia.org/wiki/Smallpox

[71]   Phillip W. Magness and Sebastian Page. *Mr. Lincoln and Mr. Johnson. The New York Times.* February 1, 2012. http://opinionator.blogs.nytimes.com/2012/02/01/mr-lincoln-and-mr-johnson/

physician would touch a patient, let alone perform a barbaric operation, in the early 1800s. One hundred years later, surgeons began operating on the brain, and surgery, while still uncommon and quite dangerous, was seen as a potentially powerful tool to address previously incurable conditions. Central to this transition was the development of effective anesthesia and an understanding of germ theory.

From the mid-1840s to the mid-1860s, the ability to block the agonizing pain of surgery through anesthesia was developed. There is considerable controversy as to who first performed successful surgery with anesthesia. One of the earliest candidates for this distinction was Horace Wells, a dentist from Hartford, CT.

On December 10th, 1844, Dr. Wells attended a traveling road show that came into town. These variety shows included a series of skits and musical performances. They often ended with a nitrous-oxide frolic. Volunteers from the audience were brought up onto the stage. They were then asked to inhale nitrous oxide from a flask. Once the nitrous oxide took effect, the volunteers would proceed to make fools of themselves, as they wandered about the stage in various states of disorientation—all to the great amusement of those in the audience. During the show, Dr. Wells witnessed Samuel Cooley, one of the audience members who had taken the nitrous oxide, stumble badly and suffer a deep gash to his leg. Dr. Wells noted with amazement that Mr. Cooley experienced essentially no pain from this injury.

Dr. Wells surmised that the use of nitrous oxide may be a benefit to his dental patients, and he sought out those who had organized the road show. The next day, he tried nitrous oxide on one of his dental patients and was amazed at how little discomfort the individual experienced when he extracted an infected tooth. Unfortunately, when he tried to replicate this anesthesia during a tooth extraction at the Massachusetts General Hospital on January 20th, 1845, the demonstration ended in failure when the patient cried out in pain. Disgraced, Wells stopped practicing as a dentist and eventually became addicted to chloroform—another anesthetic agent. He committed suicide in 1848.

In 1853, Queen Victoria demonstrated the benefits of having a celebrity endorse a treatment. She gave the fledgling anesthesia movement significant legitimacy when she allowed her physician, Dr.

John Snow, to administer chloroform during the delivery of her eighth child, Prince Leopold.[72] By the 1860s, anesthesia was still an imperfect science fraught with major complications, including death. However, it had become the norm prior to surgery. As a result, surgical technique began to overtake speed as the primary quality of a good surgeon.

The ability to have tumors or body parts removed via surgery without excruciating pain was of little benefit if the patient subsequently died of sepsis or developed a debilitating, festering chronic infection, as was the norm. Infections were so ubiquitous in surgery that surgeons of that era looked for "laudable pus." However, Louis Pasteur's identification of bacteria and subsequent promotion of the germ theory, combined with the development of antiseptic techniques by Joseph Lister during the 1870s, significantly decreased the rate of infection following surgery.

Using fine microscopes, Pasteur identified the extent of bacteria existing in the microscopic world. He correctly postulated that bacteria caused infections. He also noted that, when heated or subjected to certain chemicals, the bacteria were effectively killed. This led to "pasteurization" (heating) of milk and other perishables—a process that is still used today.

Lister, a Scottish surgeon, took Pasteur's ideas and applied them to surgery, with the goal of eradicating post-operative infections. He first proposed *antiseptic* technique—essentially killing bacteria in the surgical field as the surgery progressed. Initially he sprayed carbolic acid over the surgical field during the operation, a practice that served to decrease surgical infection rates.

In time it became apparent to Lister that *aseptic* technique was a superior approach. Aseptic surgical technique involved killing all the bacteria in the surgical field prior to an operation, and then ensuring that the operative field remained sterile throughout the surgery—by avoiding contamination from any unsterile person or surface. This approach revolutionized surgery, and aseptic technique remains the gold standard today. By the mid 1800s, with improved anesthesia techniques and the development of aseptic sterile techniques, surgery became a realistic option for treating many previously untreatable conditions.

---

[72] http://www.ph.ucla.edu/epi/snow/victoria.html

In the latter half of the 19th century, non-physicians still performed surgery. By 1900, however, all physicians had realized the potential benefits of surgery, and many had decided to train as surgeons. The era of the pioneering surgeon had begun. No body cavity, including the brain, was off limits to this new breed of physicians/surgeons. They would come to epitomize the pioneering era of medicine. Unfortunately, all too often their enthusiasm outpaced their skill, and surgical mortality remained high throughout the early part of the 20th century.

The Pioneering Era of Medicine: 1900-1999

The 20th century was an explosion of scientific discovery, including an improved understanding of disease processes and the development of numerous effective medical treatments. Many of these developments were the product of bold, strong-willed, individual physicians. Through hard work, intense dedication, and the force of their personality, individuals such as William Osler, Fredrick Banting, and John Charnley epitomized the 20th century physician.

Near where I live in San Francisco, there is a plaque dedicated to Lincoln Beachey. He was considered the most famous pilot of the early 20th century. On June 27th, 1911, he became the first person to fly over Niagara Falls. After flying over both the American and Canadian Falls, he skimmed his Curtiss biplane to within 6m of the water's surface, all to the entertainment of 150,000 cheering spectators. His loops and aeronautical acrobatics were so spectacular that in 1914, more than 17 million people—20% of the North American population—watched his flying. On March 14th, 1915, he flew his Beachey-Eaton monoplane for the first time, in front of an estimated 250,000 spectators at the San Francisco World's Fair.[73] He took the plane into an inverted loop, but when he attempted to exit this position, the strain caused the wings to break and the plane crashed into the San Francisco Bay. Like so

---

[73] Lincoln Beachey Was The Master Birdman Who Owned The Sky. http://survivor-story.com/lincoln-beachy-was-the-master-birdman-who-owned-the-sky/

many lesser pilots of the day, Lincoln Beachey, "the World's Greatest Aviator,"[74] was killed in a plane crash.

Physicians and surgeons of the early 20th century took a similar approach to their work. Pushing the boundaries of the profession was encouraged. As the public adored pilots for their daring and skill, similarly physicians' exploits were trumpeted in the newspapers of the day. However, unlike daredevil pilots, when these physicians failed, it was their patients who died.

Simultaneously, scientific advancements created expanded opportunities to improve treatments. In the early 20th century, medicine had become a glamorous, high profile, and potentially lucrative profession for many physicians and surgeons. Patients who could pay flocked to the physicians who they perceived provided the best care. Quality and effectiveness of care were associated with the individual practitioner. There was no accurate outcome data, so the reputation of the practitioner was based on perception—usually from word-of-mouth or overt marketing. Those physicians who could best differentiate themselves in a positive manner from others would receive the most patients—and by extension, the highest remuneration.

The Strong-willed Physician as Hero: The discovery of insulin

In 1919, 11-year-old Elizabeth Hughes developed the telltale signs of diabetes: excessive thirst, weight loss, and lethargy. This was the nightmare that all parents feared—a 12-18-month march to certain death for their child. Diabetes struck children of both the rich and poor with seeming randomness. Elizabeth Hughes was the daughter of one of the most powerful and well-known men in the world: Charles Evan Hughes, former United States Supreme Court Justice, Presidential candidate, and soon-to-be United States Secretary of State.

At that time, treatment of diabetes in children was not only futile, but devastating. The only thing that seemed to prolong the child's life was to essentially starve them—a strict, low-calorie, non-carbohydrate

---

[74] Marrero, Frank. *Lincoln Beachey: The Man Who Owned the Sky.* Scottwall Associates (1997) ISBN 978-0-942087-12-3.

diet. By limiting the glucose their body was exposed to, a few more months of life could be preserved. When it came, death was due to the perils of starvation, with many of the children losing close to half their body weight by the time they passed.

By religiously adhering to a strict, 500-calorie-a-day diet overseen by her physician, Dr. Frederick Allen, young Elizabeth Hughes had lived two years longer than expected. In August of 1922, she was 14 years old and weighed only 45 pounds. She could barely walk; the end was near.

It was understood that a lack of a hormone now known as insulin caused diabetes, and that this hormone was secreted by the islet cells of the pancreas. However, the pancreas had other functions, including secreting digestive enzymes, such as trypsin, into the intestinal tract. The islet cells were a relatively small part of the pancreas, and until then, it had not been possible to isolate these islet cells and the hormone they produced. Solving this puzzle led to one of the most dramatic discoveries in the history of medicine—as well as fame and notoriety for a young, headstrong Canadian physician.

On October 31, 1920, Fredrick Banting, a 28-year-old, recently-graduated physician was preparing to give a lecture at the local medical school in London, Ontario, as part of his role as a "demonstrator." The lecture was on the function of the pancreas. To prepare for the lecture, he read an article in the latest edition of *Surgery, Gynecology and Obstetrics* written by Moses Brown, a pathologist from the University of Minnesota. The article was entitled "The Relation of the Islets of Langerhans to Diabetes, With Special Reference to Cases of Pancreatic Lithiasis." The author described a case in which a calcified stone had blocked the duct of the pancreas. This blockage prevented the digestive enzymes from being secreted and caused all of the cells in the pancreas to atrophy—all of the cells except the islet cells, which were believed to secret a hormone responsible for regulating blood glucose levels.

After reading the article, Banting jotted down the following note—a note that would make medical history:

Diabetus (sic) ligate pancreatic ducts of dogs. Keep dogs alive until acini degenerate leaves islets. Try to isolate the internal secretions of these to relieve glycosurea (sic).

Beginning in May of 1921, Banting left his fledgling surgical practice in London, Ontario, to spend two months doing research in the lab of Professor John MacLeod, head of the physiology department at the University of Toronto. Charles Best—a 22-year-old, University of Toronto medical student in Professor MacLeod's lab was assigned to Banting to help him test his theory. Many dogs were sacrificed for the sake of the experiment, including some strays that were purportedly rounded up from the streets of Toronto. The dogs had their pancreatic ducts surgically ligated and after six weeks, their pancreases were harvested. These pancreases, with their concentration of insulin-producing islet cells, were then prepared in various manners in an effort to extract the blood sugar-lowering compound that the pancreas was known to produce.

Banting and his assistant Best worked long hours and suffered numerous failures. They were also naïve to research that had been performed in this area, as similar studies had already been tried and reported as being unsuccessful. However, they persevered. They noted a small success: transient lowering of the blood glucose in some of the dogs who received the pancreatic extract. They refined their technique and continued experimenting.

Professor MacLeod had spent the summer of 1921 at his family's home in Scotland. When he returned, Banting reported results that were encouraging enough to warrant a continuation of their experiments. MacLeod assigned a visiting, post-doctoral scholar named James "Bert" Collip to help improve the method of extraction.

On December 28, 1921, MacLeod reported Banting's experimental results to the American Physiology Society meeting in New Haven, CT. These preliminary results met with great interest from the diabetes experts in attendance. They called the extract they were isolating "insulin." Banting continued his obstinate pursuit of finding a pancreatic extract that would lower blood sugar in diabetics. Despite setbacks and a steadily deteriorating relationship with MacLeod, Banting with help from Best and Collip managed to improve the process to the point where they could attempt to treat humans.

Elizabeth Hughes was the fourth patient Banting treated. On August 15, 1922, Banting injected Elizabeth with her first dose of insulin. Her body responded immediately. The glucose that would normally get trapped in her blood could now be absorbed into her cells—cells that were desperate for the energy that the glucose provided. She could now eat without fear of dangerously elevating her glucose levels. Three months after starting her treatments, she left Toronto to return to her home in Washington, D.C. Elizabeth had gained more than 20 pounds and started a new life. In 1981, at the age of 73, after receiving more than 42,000 insulin injections, she passed away. Insulin was hailed as a miracle and word that a "cure" for diabetes had been found spread quickly.

Banting's approach—that of an isolated researcher toiling with his assistant to achieve a spectacular result—was the stereotypical approach to research during the 20th century, and became the norm among practicing physicians. While residency training tended to be rigid, autocratic, and focused on producing a standardized physician, once a physician was licensed, he or she was free to practice independently. Differences in approaches to treatment were not only accepted, but indirectly encouraged, so that one physician could separate their services from another's. As was the case with Banting's discovery of insulin, this independent, pioneering approach did lead to many advances in treatment. However, it also led to care that was of widely varying quality, and in many instances represented malpractice.

Banting's headstrong approach to discovering an effective treatment for diabetes was emblematic of most of the major medical discoveries of the 20th century. He was a stubborn physician who flew in the face of traditional medical conventions. He was rewarded for his stubbornness with fame and accolades, including the 1923 Nobel Prize for medicine. The government of Canada gave him a lifetime grant for research, and when he died in a plane crash in 1941, he was one of the most famous and revered Canadians.

Many other physicians and medical researchers of the 20th century followed this individualistic, stubborn model to great success. Medical advances piled up rapidly. Alexander Fleming discovered penicillin and ushered in the age of antibiotics. Drs. Jonas Salk and Albert Sabin battled viciously against each other in the 1950s—both developing an effective vaccination against the dreaded polio infection, saving countless children worldwide from the ravages of this crippling disease. Led by pioneering surgeons Dr. Michael DeBakey and Dr. Denton Cooley, open heart surgery—stopping the heart and bypassing the blood to a machine to keep it oxygenated and flowing—was developed in the 1950s. This heart bypass technique allowed for increasingly difficult heart operations to be performed, including, eventually, heart transplantations.

As more and more physicians were trained, individual practitioners with similar interests often combined to form departments within the hospitals for which they worked. The main departments stemmed from the Johns Hopkins model: surgery, medicine, gynecology, and pathology. As medicine entered the 1950s and 1960s, subspecialization increased. Cardiology, pulmonology, and neurology became subspecializations within medicine, while orthopedics, urology, and neurosurgery were now subspecialties within the surgical disciplines.

As the number of subspecialists grew, separate departments broke off from medicine and surgery to house these subspecialists. At the time, it may have seemed logical to segment the profession according to the personal interests of various physicians; after all, the profession was largely made up of independent physician practitioners. However, this segmentation due to *physician specialization* —rather than by the *patient conditions* —eventually led to ensconced silos. This created fragmentation within the medical system, which has now proven prohibitively difficult to overcome.

Typical of the pioneering spirit among physicians was English surgeon John Charnley's development of the first effective total hip replacement. Arthritis of the hip joint is an all too common problem. As certain individuals age, excessive loading from uneven wear across the hip joint can lead to a destruction of the cartilage within the joint. This creates a painful limping gait that is debilitating for the patients. The condition has been known for over 100 years, but by the 1950s, there was still no effective surgical treatment. Some surgeons recommended cutting out the hip joint itself. This method did improve pain, but led to a markedly abnormal gait, and subsequently to pain in the back and knees.

Faced with this clinical problem, John Charnley set about designing and developing a hip replacement in the 1950s. After multiple experiments, he began piecing together the elements of what would eventually become a successful hip replacement. He determined that the replacement should have a cup that fits into the socket (acetabulum) of the hip joint; a stem that extended down into the thigh bone (femur); and, perhaps most importantly, a low-friction interface between the two. The first low-friction surface he tried was polytetrafluorethylene, also known as Teflon®.

From 1958-1962, Charnley inserted his new hip replacement with Teflon as the bearing surface in over 300 patients. After short-term, spectacular successes, almost all of these hip replacements failed and needed to be removed. The Teflon bearing surface wore down quickly and caused marked tissue reaction around the hip joint. He next tried high-molecular-weight polyethylene as a bearing surface, which proved to be much more successful.

However, Charnley soon noted that infections were becoming increasingly common in his surgeries, and when they occurred, this complication was devastating. He systematically developed a process to minimize the risk of infection, which included adding antibiotics to the bone cement that was used as grout to secure the prosthesis. This process, combined with meticulous sterile technique and a sterile, positive-pressure, air-filtration system within the operating room, succeeded in lowering the deep infection rate to acceptable levels.

By the late 1960s, Charnley had addressed many of the early problems associated with total hip replacement, and his clinical results were good. Surgeons came from all over the world to learn the Charnley method of total hip replacement. By the early 1970s, the hip replacements that John Charnley performed would prove to be so successful that his long-term results have yet to be surpassed. These results are a testament to Charnley's strength of will. He tackled this problem largely alone, fighting through resistance from the hospital staff and fellow physicians. He never gave up, despite multiple spectacular failures. He was tireless in his pursuit of this goal, and today, patients with arthritic hips are benefactors of this iron-willed dedication.

Charnley's development of an effective total hip replacement in the 1950s and 1960s was emblematic of the explosion of new surgical and medical treatments. In the latter half of the 20th century, at least 75% of the orthopaedic procedures that are commonly performed today either did not exist or were not widely performed prior to 1970.

At the same time Charnley was introducing the hip replacement to the world, a variety of knee replacements were introduced by pioneering surgeons. Canadian Dr. Bob Jackson introduced arthroscopy to North America. During a visit to Japan in the 1960s, Dr. Masaki Watanabe taught him the technique of inserting a small scope into a joint. He started performing the procedure in Toronto and steadily perfected the ability to correct problems within the knee and other joints, saving the careers of countless athletes. Arthroscopy is now the most common orthopaedic procedure in North America, and in 1994, Dr. Jackson was named one of the 40 most influential men in sports by *Sports Illustrated*.

Beginning in the 1950s, Dr. Paul Harrington developed an innovative approach to stabilizing spine deformities by surgically placing a *Harrington rod* in the back. Prior to this, a patient having his or her spine fused needed to spend months in a cast, and often suffered non-unions and recurrence of the deformity. The development of Harrington rods—and subsequently, other means of instrumented spinal fusion—revolutionized spinal care and created an explosion in the number of spinal surgeries performed.

Maurice Mueller and Martin Allgower helped form the AO group[75], based in Switzerland and dedicated to the surgical treatment of fractures. The resulting discoveries completely changed the way fractures were treated. As the "AO principles" caught on in the 1960s and '70s, patients who would have previously spent months lying in traction while their thigh bones healed could now be up and moving about in days. Joint replacements, joint arthroscopy, instrumented spinal fusions, and internal fixation of fractures were all developed in the '50s

---

[75]   AO stands for *Arbeitsgemeinschaft für Osteosynthesefragen*. In English, this group is know as the *Association for the Study of Internal Fixation*.

and '60s and optimized in the '70s and '80s, fundamentally altering the practice of orthopaedics.

These types of revolutionary developments in the latter half of the 20th century were not confined to orthopaedics. Chemotherapeutic regiments and bone marrow transplantations were developed to cure leukemia and other previously-incurable cancers. Powerful antibiotics were developed to eradicate or control previously deadly infections. The discovery of new drugs and innovative multi-drug treatment regiments lead to successful long-term management of human immunodeficiency virus (HIV) infections. Similarly, medications were developed to effectively control blood pressure and therefore improve longevity. Treatments, many of them highly effective, were developed in all aspects of medicine.

Since 1900, 20th century medicine has transformed itself from a discipline with only a handful of effective treatments to a profession with effective (although not necessarily curative) treatments for almost every ailment—and a highly-trained and tightly-regulated physician and nursing workforce. This is what the world of medicine looked like in the 1990s. However, two inescapable facts were emerging, and once these facts became widely known, they led to the natural conclusion that medicine needed to fundamentally reform itself. Thus began a new era in medicine.

The Era of Systematized Medical Care: 2000–Present

Two realities had emerged from the *pioneering era of medicine* in the 20th century:

1. Medical care was highly variable.
2. Many patients were being unnecessarily harmed by the existing system.

In 1996 researchers at Dartmouth University started the *Dartmouth Atlas of Healthcare* to map variations in healthcare delivery in the United

States, based on hard data.[76,77] Updated yearly, the *Atlas* notes staggering variations in practice patterns—not merely 2-5% differences, but 100-200% differences or more for many common treatments.

This was not just an American problem. Studies examining the Canadian healthcare system also showed wide variation in treatment practices, especially among elective surgeries or treatments.[78] These differences were based on where the care was delivered and which physician was in charge of the patient. This marked variation in care delivery was problematic. Decreasing variation is one of the established hallmarks of a high-performing "production system"—a principle that had been worked out via the quality and process improvement movement, which had taken place in other industries, including airlines, automobile manufacturing, and hotel service.[79,80]

The second fact that emerged is that the medical system that evolved during the 20th century harms many patients. Being admitted to a hospital can be dangerous to your health. Two large, high-quality research studies in the 1990s demonstrated that significant errors impacted between 6.6 and 13.4% of hospitalized patients. Incorrect medications were given, patients acquired infections caused by the hospital itself, tests were ordered but not checked with catastrophic results, and the wrong operation was performed on the wrong patient or the wrong extremity. These types of medical systems errors were pervasive.

---

[76]   http://www.dartmouthatlas.org/pages/variation_surgery_2

[77]   http://www.vox.com/2014/9/18/6251063/
       health-care-waste-dartmouth-atlas-sheiner

[78]   Gentleman, J.F., Vayda, E., Parsons, G.F., and Walsh, M.N. Surgical rates
       in subprovincial areas across Canada: rankings of 39 procedures in order of
       variation. Can J Surg. Oct 1996; 39(5): 361–367.

[79]   *What is the Law of Variation?* American Society for Quality Website Based
       on Timothy J. Clark, *Success Through Quality: Support Guide for the Journey
       to Continuous Improvement*, ASQ Quality Press, 1999. (http://asq.org/learn-
       about-quality/variation/overview/overview.html accessed April 28th, 2015)

[80]   Deming's 14 key principles from *Out of the Crisis* by W. Edwards
       Deming. Cambridge, Mass.: Massachusetts Institute of Technology,
       Center for Advanced Engineering Study, ©1986. (*http://en.wikipedia.org/
       wiki/W._Edwards_Deming accessed April 28th 2015*)

The percentage of patients affected may have been low, but given the sheer volume of patients that were now being hospitalized, the number of individuals suffering complications, including death, was staggering. In 1999, the *Institute of Medicine* estimated that between 44,000 and 98,000 people were killed each year by medical errors in the United States.[81] This meant that if *medical error* was an official cause of death, it would be either the 8th or 5th leading cause of death in the United States.

The most striking element of all of these complications was that they were, in theory, easily preventable. Double-check the medications given to patients to ensure they are receiving the correct medication, the correct dose, and the correct route. Wash your hands between patients, so germs are not spread between patients by nurses and doctors. Actually look at the blood test, urine test, or x-ray you ordered, so that if signs of cancer or other serious illness are identified, early treatment can be instituted. Check to ensure the correct operation is being performed on the correct patient.

Conceptually, these errors should *never* have happened, yet they occur with frightening regularity within the medical systems led by doctors from the pioneering era of medicine. Humans make mistakes. This was the price the medical system and patients were paying for relying on individuals.

How many commercial airline pilots do you know? Perhaps you remember Sully Sullenberger, who dramatically landed US Airways Flight 1549 in the Hudson River on January 15, 2009, after both engines failed. However, if you are like most people, you don't know any commercial airline pilots, and that is exactly the way the airlines want it to be; after all, notoriety in the industry is usually preceded by a catastrophic event. Daring, fearless, and experimental were terms used to describe Lincoln Beachey and his fellow pilots a hundred years ago. Today, you would be right to run in fear if you knew such an individual was piloting the airplane you were traveling on. Modern airline pilots are expected to be experienced, professional, and systematic.

---

[81] Committee on Quality of Health Care in America, Institute of Medicine. *To Err is Human: Building a Safer Health System. Washington, DC: Institute of Medicine*; 2000. p. 1

According to Atul Gawande in his book *The Checklist Manifesto*, the nature of piloting fundamentally changed on October 30, 1935, when the US government was trialing planes for a large military contract. Boeing had the contract virtually secured. Their plane, the Model 299, was bigger, faster, and more fuel-efficient than the rival planes from Douglas and Martin. However, as the massive Boeing plane took off, it became apparent that it was not gaining height. It crashed, killing two of the crewmembers, including legendary test pilot Major Ployer "Pete" Hill. Boeing lost the contract, and the company almost went bankrupt.

The cause of the crash was not mechanical failure. The pilot, Major Hill, simply forgot to release the flaps, and the drag caused the plane to crash. It was a fundamental but deadly mistake. It would have been easy to blame the pilot and move on. However, Major Hill was universally regarded as an outstanding pilot. If he could make such a mistake, any pilot could. Among the hundreds of things he needed to do in order for the plane to take off successfully, he had forgotten only one, and it had killed him.

The plane was deemed "too much for one man to fly." Flying this engineering marvel required a different approach. The Federal Aviation Administration (FAA) recommended that from this point forward, flying needed to be much more systematic. Today, pilots and mechanics use checklists to ensure all steps have been performed appropriately. Every pilot is tested extensively, using flight simulators to ensure they have experience handling almost any situation they may encounter. When they do occur, problems are systematically analyzed, and the results of these analyses are quickly disseminated to all of the airlines and commercial pilots throughout the world. The result is that traveling by plane is now the safest form of transportation.

In the average hospital, 0.28% of patients will die directly or indirectly from medical errors.[82] If the airlines had the same error rate, there would be 80 commercial plane crashes every day in North

---

[82] There are 35.1 million patients hospitalized each year in the United States (http://www.cdc.gov/nchs/fastats/hospital.htm). With an estimated 98,000 unnecessary deaths based on the studies by …..., this leads to an unnecessary death rate of 0.28%.

America.[83] There is much that the medical systems can learn from the aviation industry.

If you need your shoulder fixed, don't go there. If you need thyroid surgery, don't go there. But if you need your hernia fixed, *The Shouldice Clinic* in Thornhill, Ontario, is the best place in the world to be. All they do is fix hernias. Founded in 1945 by Dr. Edward Shouldice, the entire organization is focused on providing the highest level of care for patients with hernias.

Like the start of the *pioneering era* one hundred years earlier, the seeds of change started in the previous century. Thus it is that institutions focused on excellence in coordinated, team-based care— such as the Shouldice clinic—have provided a roadmap for delivering care in the era of *systematized practice*. Concentrated excellence, a team-based approach, continuous quality improvement, and a relentless focus on outcomes are all hallmarks of systematized medical care.

To the outside observer, the Canadian healthcare system should be ideally set up to provide the type of high-quality, organized care that is characteristic of the era of *systematized practice*. All patients have insurance covering physician and hospital expenses. Furthermore, it is the same insurance, thereby allowing a free flow of patients to local and regional centers of excellence (at least within each province).

Most importantly, there is central oversight of the system that should allow for the establishment of these types of coordinated programs. The natural evolution of the practice of medicine, as outlined in this chapter, demands that the model of care delivery needs to fundamentally change. However, as will be illustrated in the next chapter, the historical basis that established the framework of the existing Canadian healthcare system precludes this type of meaningful coordination.

Summary: Chapter 4

Like professional hockey players, the skills associated with individual physicians have improved exponentially in the past hundred years.

---

[83]   There are an average of 28,537 commercial flights each day in North America (http://sos.noaa.gov/Datasets/dataset.php?id=44). If 0.28% of these flights crashed, there would be 80 crashes.

Physicians and hockey players routinely perform maneuvers today that would have been unimaginable a hundred years ago (or even fifty years ago). These individual qualities are a product of improvements in equipment, training methodology, and the wisdom of experience.

Hockey has always been a team sport with individual stars. However, after the 1972 Soviet Summit series, players, coaches, and fans began to see what it meant to really play as a team. Today, every manager and coach of a professional hockey team knows their team must play as a highly-integrated and coordinated unit to have any chance of winning consistently. We now know that for optimal success, the same principle is true for medicine.

Unlike hockey, where performance results are there for everyone to observe, hard, accurate outcome data has traditionally been less forthcoming in medicine. As a result, there has not been the same pressure to move physicians and healthcare administrators away from the individual-oriented, physician-dominated, pioneering era of medicine. This is changing as outcome measures emerge as one of the cornerstones of modern medicine. Likewise, a new era of healthcare is emerging—the era of team-oriented *systematized practice*.

Summary Points: Chapter 4

To envision the medical system of the future, it is critical to understand how the delivery of medical care has evolved.

Medicine can be viewed as having three broad eras:

1) the *era of magical thinking* (pre 1900),
2) the *pioneering era* (1900-2000), and
3) the *era of systematized care delivery* (post 2000).

The *era of magical thinking* was characterized by physicians who had little formal training and rendered treatment that was often of limited effectiveness.

The *pioneering era* saw strong-willed, independent physicians generate an explosion of scientific discoveries, including an improved understanding of disease processes and the development of numerous effective medical treatments.

Two realities emerged from the *pioneering era of medicine* at the end of the 20th century:

1. Medical care was markedly variable, often by 200+%.
2. Many patients were unnecessarily harmed by the existing healthcare system.

These findings lead to the inescapable conclusion that the system needed to be fundamentally reformed. This created the impetus to usher in the *era of systematized care delivery*, characterized by coordinated team-based care that focuses on measuring and optimizing each patient's ultimate outcome.

CHAPTER 5

Trapped by History: A Historical Perspective on the Canadian Medical System

The organization of hockey, including the rules by which the game is played, has evolved considerably since the 1890s. Early hockey players were amateurs. However, as the popularity of the sport increased, many team owners were making large sums of money selling tickets. Naturally, this did not sit well with many of the players.

When Canadian Jack Gibson formed the Michigan-based International Hockey League (IHL) in 1904, hockey had its first professional league. This league drew many talented players from Ontario and other parts of Canada. In 1907, the Ontario Professional Hockey League (OPHL) was formed to compete against the IHL.

Professional hockey players in the early 1900s were true free agents. Many of the early professional games were exhibition matches, played in front of thousands of paying spectators, and players were usually paid on a per-game basis. Most players made decisions based on their individual goals— often choosing to play for whichever teams paid them the most money.

When competing professional hockey leagues—such as the IHL and OPHL, and later, the Canadian Hockey Association (CHA) and rival National Hockey Association (NHA)—were formed, team owners regularly raided players from other leagues by paying them more money. It was not uncommon for players to move between teams in various leagues, even in the midst of a season. To help stem this problem and encourage a more stable team environment, owners began signing players to season-long contracts. Still, defections were not uncommon, as players sought more lucrative opportunities.

In 1917, after more than a decade of the forming and disbanding of various professional leagues, the National Hockey League was organized as the successor to the NHA. Although other competing professional leagues, including the American Hockey League and the Pacific Coast Hockey League, still existed, the NHL eventually became the primary place of employment for professional hockey players. Those running the fledgling NHL focused on team stability and performance, realizing that high-quality teams playing an exciting brand of hockey would increase the number of paying fans.

Just as early hockey underwent a dramatic restructuring of the way teams and leagues were organized, the rules of hockey also underwent marked change. Early hockey games were played with seven players per team on the ice. No substitutions were allowed, except in the case of injury. Prior to 1910, the game consisted of two 30-minute halves, so player fatigue often played a major factor in games.

In order to increase the speed of play and improve the excitement of the game for fans, the NHA changed the rules to allow substitutions in 1911.[85] Simultaneously, they decreased the number of players on the ice to six, standardizing the positions to include one goaltender, two defensemen, and three forwards—eliminating the position of rover.

The early rules of hockey made forward passes illegal. Players either shot the puck into the opposing team's end and raced after it, or they had a single player carry the puck toward the other team's net in an attempt to score. Gradually, forward passes were legalized—first within the neutral zone in the middle of the ice in 1918, then in the defensive end in 1927, and finally in the offensive zone in 1929. Allowing forward passes in all three zones increased the offense and the excitement of the game by encouraging more coordinated, team-oriented play.

---

[84]   http://www.rauzulusstreet.com/hockey/nhlhistory/nhlrules.html

To discourage certain behaviours, such as tripping and slashing, penalties were introduced. Penalties were standardized in 1918 by sending offending players off the ice for 3 minutes for minor infractions (reduced to 2 minutes in 1921), and for 5 minutes for major infractions. During this time, no substitutions for the offending player were allowed—meaning his team played at a one-man disadvantage.

The rules of hockey continue to evolve even today—albeit not with the same dramatic changes that occurred prior to 1930. In 1991, the NHL added video replays to help determine whether a puck had crossed the goal line. In 2010, a mandatory concussion protocol was introduced to help ensure the longer-term health of the players by preventing a premature return to playing after a concussion.[86]

Hockey has always involved intense competition between teams. However, modern team owners realize that when the league as a whole does well, they all do well. Rule changes have been introduced with the goal of directly or indirectly increasing the excitement, fairness, and safety of the game. This serves to improve the satisfaction of the fans, and thereby increase the popularity of the sport.

---

[85] http://sportsdocuments.com/nhl-protocol-for-concussion-evaluation-and-management/

Introduction

The Canadian healthcare system is a prisoner of its history. To understand the ills of the present-day healthcare system, one needs to understand how it came to be formed. It is akin to a large sprawling house built without a solid foundation. The structural organization of the healthcare system was set at the time of its formation. However, what we now call the healthcare system was never designed as a system. It developed piece by piece—first as a means to fund hospital care in the late 1950s; a decade later, funding of physician services was added. Other essential aspects of an integrated health system such as a comprehensive drug plan and long-term care have never been added.

The Canadian "healthcare system," unlike the British National Health Service, is about funding specific fragments of medical care—not developing and coordinating an integrated healthcare system. As this chapter will assert, the historical shackles inherent in this piecemeal structure served to create most of the problems we see today.

Canadian Healthcare in the 1800s

Canada's first prime minister, Sir John A. Macdonald, died a fairly typical death for a middle-class or upper-class Canadian in the 1800s. On March 5, 1891, after a hard campaign during which McDonald fell ill, his conservative government was returned to power, and he was elected Prime Minister for the sixth time.

The campaign had taken its toll on the 76-year-old statesman. He began to recover somewhat from the demands of the campaign, but on May 23, 1891, he suffered a stroke, causing partial paralysis. Had this happened today, he would have been rushed to the hospital, undergone a CT scan, and then been treated with thrombolysis to break down the clot in an attempt to minimize the damage to his brain caused by the stroke. However, in 1891, there were no effective treatments. So he rested and tried to resume his work, and his personal physician, Dr. R.W. Powell, attended to him regularly at his home in Earnscliffe Manor, Ottawa.

Six days later, on Friday, May 29, he suffered a massive stroke from which he never recovered.[86] He was speechless and entirely paralyzed on the right side. Dr. Powell attended to him daily, attempting to make him comfortable. News bulletins were issued regularly to update the public. Canada's first prime minister died in his home eight days later on June 6, 1891. In many ways this was a normal death in the 1800s. Being treated at your home in the company of your family, with care from a personal physician, was the norm for those who could afford it.

In the 1800s, and for much of the early part of the 20th century, hospitals were largely for the poor. They did not offer much in the way of effective treatment. Often, the disease and bacteria present in the hospitals made patients worse. Most hospitals built in the 1800s were done so through the auspices of religious organizations—with the goal of providing comfortable care and religious support to the poor in their time of sickness.

In 1843 the Most Reverend Ignace Bourget, Bishop of Montreal, established the Daughters of Charity Servants of the Poor under the leadership of Mother Emilie Gamelin.[87] This order of nuns was dedicated to providing service and care to the poor, elderly, and orphaned, and it soon became known as the Sisters of Providence.[88] They formed local orphanages, developed care homes for elderly women, and established charity hospitals.

Beginning in 1852, small groups of sisters from this order were sent forth to establish hospitals throughout Canada, the Pacific Northwest, and other parts of the world.[89] This was done as a service to the Catholic Church and, over a number of decades, led to the development of numerous charity hospitals. Subsequently, a large chain of Catholic hospitals was established, eventually becoming one of the largest hospital chains in North America. Many faith-based hospitals still exist today.

This illustration of providing relief from suffering for the poor, administered by a religious organization, was typical of the 1800s. Hospitals served a critical function in caring for the poor and needy.

---

[86] Newman, Lena. The John A MacDonald Album. Tundra Books Inc. 1974.

[87] http://www.providencehealthcare.org/hospitals-residences/st-pauls-hospital/overview/history

[88] http://www.providenceintl.org/en/

[89] http://sistersofprovidence.net/150years/index.php?page=history&h=timeline

However, the effectiveness of the medical care that these hospitals provided was limited by the lack of understanding of disease processes that existed during that time.

In the 19th century, it was common for well-to-do members of society to support charity hospitals. However, it was not common for them to receive care at these hospitals. Most medical care provided to the middle and upper classes was delivered in their homes or at their local physician's offices. Physicians who had widely varying skills and training would set up independent practices in a community and attempt to attract patients, who would in turn pay them for the care they provided. This was commonly a fee-for-service transaction. Occasionally, patients who could not afford care would provide service *in kind* for treatment (i.e., in lieu of payment).

In an effort to offset high costs that were incurred in the course of acute or chronic illnesses, rudimentary health insurance plans were established. They were often coordinated through the workplace. These insurance plans helped more evenly distribute the cost of healthcare, but they still recognized and fostered the individual nature of each physician's practice, as well as their right to charge the fees they felt were appropriate.

The British Parliament passed the *British North America Act* (BNA) of 1867, which established the federal Dominion of Canada and set up the framework for the new government. The *BNA Act* was subsequently revised multiple times, and in 1982, it was revised once again and renamed the *Constitution Act*. In addition to setting up the House of Commons, senate, and judicial system, the *BNA of 1867* delineated the responsibilities of the federal and provincial governments.

The *BNA Act* dealt with healthcare using the framework of that day and age.[90] Many people in the 1860s died of infections, particularly tuberculosis, which was felt to be caused or related to decay and filth. Therefore, healthcare was more about keeping cities clean than actually treating illnesses. In this era before germ theory, surgery, and antibiotics, most illnesses did not have effective, science-based treatments. The *BNA*

---

[90] "Cracks in the Foundations: The Origins of the Canadian and American Health Care Systems" (Chapter 10), p. 269. From *Staying Alive: Critical Perspectives on Health, Illness, and Health Care*. Edited by Dennis Raphael, Toba Bryant, Marcia H. Rioux.

Act of 1867 assigned oversight of quarantines and marine hospitals to the federal government. To the provincial governments, they assigned the local jurisdiction of healthcare (i.e., sanitation). This is why oversight of healthcare today is a provincial rather than a federal jurisdiction.

Canadian Healthcare in the Early 1900s

In the early 20th century, effective treatments, particularly with respect to surgery, became more common. X-ray machines were introduced, advances in operative techniques and anesthesia led to improved surgical results, and many hospitals installed modern operating room facilities. As a result, more and more citizens began receiving care at their local hospitals. Many hospitals responded to this increase in paying middle and upper class patients by establishing private hospital wings separate from the area where charity care was provided. These private wings served as an additional source of revenue for the hospital and often helped to fund the hospital's overall budget.

Canada's participation in the Great War, now known as World War I, was instrumental in planting the seeds of a national healthcare system. A generation of young Canadian men served alongside the British and other Allied forces during World War I. The toll, in terms of injuries and death, was staggering—almost 65,000 Canadians killed in action, and over 170,000 troops injured.[91,92]

In addition, between 30,000 and 50,000 Canadians died from the Spanish Flu epidemic of 1918. This epidemic was estimated to have killed 100 million people worldwide—more deaths than were incurred in World War I.[93] Canadian soldiers fighting in the war received medical treatment for their injuries and illnesses, as part of their service as soldiers.

When they returned to Canada, the general public rightly expected this group of heroic young men to have their medical needs met. Programs were set up through the Canadian Armed Forces to ensure that a baseline

---

[91]   The Commonwealth War Graves Commission Annual Report 2010-2011, Page 45

[92]   http://www.canadaatwar.ca/content-8/world-war-i/facts-and-information/

[93]   http://www.thestar.com/life/health_wellness/2008/09/19/ spanish_flu_killed_millions_but_few_remember.html

level of medical care was provided to these injured soldiers. Out of this experience developed a growing sentiment among the population—that the Canadian government could provide its citizens with basic medical care. This view among the public percolated for many years, eventually culminating in the introduction of Medicare in 1968.

The first example of a national healthcare program in Canada was based on sound ideas, which present-day governments could learn from. They created a coordinated program that was focused on the treatment and prophylaxis of a specific condition. In 1920, venereal disease was rampant among Canadians. Returning soldiers from World War I, a marked increase in geographic movement of the population within Canada, and the lack of effective treatments led to an epidemic of sexually transmitted infections (STIs).

In an effort to reverse this trend, the Canadian government gave annual, conditional grants of around $200,000, beginning in 1920, to fund the Canadian National Council for Combating Venereal Diseases (later renamed the Canadian Social Hygiene Council in 1922). This money allowed for the establishment of venereal disease clinics in each province except for Prince Edward Island—52 clinics in total.[94] The federal government provided the money, but jurisdiction and organization of the clinics was run provincially.

Canadian Healthcare During the Depression and World War II

Canada is a massive country, the second largest by landmass of any nation in the world. From its conception in 1867 through the 1920s and '30s, it remained sparsely populated outside of the metropolitan areas of eastern Canada. Disparate groups in a variety of different communities took on the challenge of providing healthcare to the population in various ways. Commissions were formed, studies were performed, and discussions ensued in various legislatures.

However, no widespread, sustained healthcare reform was instituted during this time. The medical profession continued to improve its capacity to treat the sick and injured, although the quality of care

---

[94]   Ch. 3.8, *This is Public Health: A Canadian History.* C Rutty and S Sullivan, 2010.

was still widely variable and largely ineffective by today's standards. Doctors continued to promote their autonomy and individuality. Fee-for-service compensation was the norm. This became problematic for many physicians when an increasingly large percentage of the population was unable to pay for these services.

The Depression hit Canada in the 1930s and devastated the country economically, including its physicians. Many physicians could no longer make a living when most of their patients were unable to pay for the care they provided. General practitioners in British Columbia saw their income drop by 36% from 1929 to 1933, and more than half of the physicians in Hamilton could not meet their operating expenses the same year.[95,96]

In 1930, Manitoba doctors went on strike, demanding some government compensation for treatment of the uninsured. Doctors in Saskatchewan also suffered tremendously. Some were able to convince local communities to hire them. Others received government support to allow them to continue in their practice. Many other physicians left the province or took up a different profession.

The harsh financial reality of the 1930s spurred a movement among doctors to have their services paid for via government coffers. In 1934, the Economic Committee of the Canadian Medical Association (CMA) drew up a plan to create a nationalized health insurance scheme that would cover both hospital and physician services. The CMA membership adopted this proposal in 1942. This was a clear illustration of the general support among Canadian physicians of that era for a government-run health plan. The CMA remained officially supportive of a national healthcare system until 1949—when circumstances changed, and they reversed their position.[97]

---

95   Ostry, Alex. "Health Care Financing to World War II" (Ch. 1) p 22 in *Change and Continuity in Canada's Health Care System.* CHA Press. 2006.

96   Gagan, D. and R Gagan. *For Patients of Moderate Means: A Social history of the Voluntary general hospital in Canada, 1890-1950.* Montreal: McGill-Queen's University Press, 2002.

97   Taylor MG, Stevenson M, Williams P. *Medical Perspectives on Canadian Medicare: Attitudes of Canadian Physicians to Policies and Problems of the Medical Care insurance Program.* Toronto: Institute for Behavioural Research, 1984.

The Depression created a crisis, but this did not lead to an immediate solution to Canada's healthcare problems. However, the ideas and passions that flowed from this era had a profound effect on the development of the Canadian healthcare system.

One such effect was the formation and popularization of the *Cooperative Commonwealth Federation* (CCF), a left-wing socialist organization committed to social reform. This party gained popularity in Saskatchewan and other western provinces. The formation of the CCF in 1932 was, in many respects, a response to the perception that capitalism had failed the people during the Depression. The CCF party's agenda promoted widespread social reforms, including "a completely socialized health service under the control and direction of the provincial governments."[98] In the aftermath of the Depression, the CCF flourished.

Canada's entrance into World War II produced the economic stimulation the country needed. Once again large numbers of Canadian soldiers headed overseas to fight on behalf of the Allied forces—and once again their healthcare needs were fully provided for during their combat years.

In Britain during the height of the war, a report was commissioned by the British government and delivered by Lord Beveridge. He proposed a broad safety net for the people, including a national health plan. Many elements contained in this report were subsequently incorporated into the *National Health Service* (NHS), which was formed by the British parliament on July 5, 1948. The NHS program was intended to be a true, coordinated health service—not merely a way to fund health care. Physicians and hospitals that were part of the NHS were not merely funded, but were given specific roles and responsibilities in support of providing the necessary care required by the population at large. The NHS offered universal healthcare to all British citizens, and it became a model for many in Canada who favored a coordinated, socialized healthcare system.

This group included Tommy Douglas. Born in Scotland in 1904, Douglas injured his knee and developed a chronic bone infection prior to leaving Scotland with his family in 1919. They initially moved to Winnipeg, where his infection flared up. It looked as if he would need

---

[98] *Social Planning for Canada.* League for Social Reconstruction.

to have his leg amputated. However, Dr. R.J. Smith, a well-respected, local surgeon, agreed to treat him for no charge, provided his parents allowed medical students to be involved in his care.[99] After a number of surgeries, Douglas's infection was controlled, and his leg was saved.

The events had a profound effect on young Tommy Douglas. He later stated: "I felt that no boy should have to depend, either for his leg or his life, upon the ability of his parents to raise enough money to bring a first-class surgeon to his bedside."[100] In 1930, Douglas graduated from Brandon College and was ordained as a Baptist minister. During the Depression, he observed the critical need for extensive social reform in Canada. He became politically active, pushing for increased government involvement in providing a safety net for its citizens. Douglas was elected to Canada's House of Parliament in 1935 and subsequently became the leader of Saskatchewan's CCF party in 1942 and provincial Premier in 1944.

Canadian Healthcare in the 1950s and '60s

By the early 1950s, the provision of medical care in Canada looked dramatically different than the care Sir John A MacDonald had experienced 60 years earlier. The number of hospitals had grown tremendously, and they were now filled with patients from all socioeconomic backgrounds. In many instances, hospitalization offered significantly improved treatment from the in-home care that had been the norm. Sterile technique and anesthesia had dramatically improved, thereby making many surgical operations routine. Penicillin was discovered in 1928 by Alexander Fleming, who was subsequently awarded the 1945 Nobel Prize in Medicine. Antibiotics such as penicillin offered potentially effective treatment for many serious infections that had been invariably fatal a generation earlier.

As Canada entered the second half of the 20th century, there were still many unknowns in medicine. However, physicians now offered

---

[99] http://www.historymuseum.ca/cmc/exhibitions/hist/medicare/medic-3g03e.shtml

[100] Lewis H. Thomas, ed. *The Making of a Socialist: The Recollections of T. C. Douglas.* Edmonton: University of Alberta Press, 1982, p. 7.

numerous effective treatments. Physician training had become more standardized and rigorous, but once trained, physician autonomy and independence had become ingrained in the system. Each physician was their own entity, free to decide how best to treat their individual patients.

With their increasing effectiveness and a booming post-World War II economy, most physicians were now doing quite well financially. This caused widespread resistance to socialized medicine among the physician population in Canada. Whereas for the previous generation the CMA had supported socialized medicine, they changed their policy in 1949 and no longer supported this form of healthcare provision.

During the 1950s, hospitals became the primary location for the management of serious (and some non-serious) medical and surgical problems. The number of hospitals and hospital beds increased dramatically. Most physicians obtained *hospital privileges*—admitting their patients to hospital and overseeing their care.

The federal government, looking to support healthcare within the country, introduced the *Hospital Insurance and Diagnostic Services (HIDS) Act* in 1957. This act guaranteed that the federal government would match provincial funding for the costs of inpatient and outpatient hospital services—to ensure that individual Canadians would not be required to pay the high cost of hospitalization. By matching provincial contributions, the act had the unintended consequence of discouraging *user fees* (although not prohibiting them), as the federal government would not match fees paid by the patient toward the cost of their hospitalization.

An additional effect of the *HIDS Act* was the growth of hospitals and hospital beds in Canada. This led to a dominant position for hospitals, as well as the funding they received within the healthcare system. This hospital-centered funding model remains intact today, although the means by which care is delivered has changed dramatically.

An analysis by Alec Ostry in his book, *Change and Continuity in Canada's Health Care System*, outlines the implications of passage of the HIDS Act by the Federal government:

> *"A major limitation of the national hospital insurance legislation was that services were only insured if delivered*

in a hospital by a physician. Outpatient services delivered in a doctor's office were not covered initially. Nor were services provided in other locations such as provincial mental hospitals, at home, or in nursing homes. This limitation of the 1957 hospital insurance plan profoundly shaped the subsequent evolution of the Canadian health system into one that is still mainly hospital based and physician centered. This factor has proven to be an enduring barrier to health system reform."[101]

Once built, hospitals were owned and run by the respective provincial governments. The hospitals provided a physical structure—the healthcare playing field. However, like a hockey arena, hospitals required personnel in order to function. Physicians were funded via a fee-for-service method or patients' insurance programs.

However, essentially all other hospital personnel—nurses, physical therapists, cleaning staff, maintenance workers, and administrators—were employed, directly or indirectly, by the government-funded hospitals. To cover the wages and salaries of these individuals, funding was generally provided via annual bulk grants to each of the hospitals from the provincial government, which in return received federal funding via the *HIDS Act*. Employees worked to keep each hospital functioning, while the admitting physicians practiced their own individualized care to the patients they had admitted to the hospital.

This model likely made sense when it was introduced in the 1950s; patient care was clearly under the jurisdiction of each admitting physician. However, in subsequent decades as the provision of medical care transitioned to a team-based concept, this model of separating physician funding (and responsibility) from the other members of the healthcare team became increasingly problematic.

It was into this environment of medicine and healthcare that the CCF, under Tommy Douglas's leadership, pushed their social reform agenda. First elected into power in 1944, the CCF (later renamed the New Democratic Party) ruled Saskatchewan for decades. In 1960, the

---

[101]   Alec Ostry. *Change and Continuity in Canada's Health Care System.* CHA Press, Ottawa 2006, p. 42.

Douglas-led CCF party was reelected for a fifth time, winning 37 of 54 seats. Their campaign platform had included the introduction of socialized medicine and they took their majority victory as a mandate to introduce such a program. In 1961, Tommy Douglas left the party to serve as leader of the recently-formed federal New Democratic Party, in an effort to expand these ideas to the national level.

Woodrow Lloyd succeeded Douglas as Saskatchewan Premier in 1961. That year, under Lloyd's leadership, the CCF introduced a proposal for socialized medicine. It met with staunch resistance from the physicians of Saskatchewan. Undaunted, the CCF pushed forward. This precipitated a 23-day doctor strike, starting on July 1, 1962. Physicians were adamant that they would not come under the financial and regulatory oversight of the Saskatchewan provincial government.

Initially, it appeared that the doctors had strong support from the business community and much of the general public. However, after almost two weeks of striking, it became apparent that the silent majority in Saskatchewan actually supported the government's move to introduce socialized medicine. Eventually, the doctors capitulated and negotiated a concession for indirect government payment. They would still be paid on a fee-for-service basis, but with the government as the source of funding. Saskatchewan had socialized medical care for the entire province, and this became a blueprint for the rest of Canada.

At the same time that Saskatchewan introduced socialized medicine to Canada, the federal government started on an inauspicious path, which ultimately led to permanent changes to the healthcare system. The Progressive Conservative Party, under Prime Minister John Diefenbaker, was elected with a minority government in 1957, and was then reelected with the largest majority in Canadian history in 1958. They were a right-of-center, pro-business party that had expressed no meaningful opinions on government-run healthcare. As such, they were seen as an ally of Canada's physicians.

In 1961, the Canadian Medical Association (CMA), sensing that they would have a supportive ear in their quest to prevent socialized medicine spreading outside of Saskatchewan, formally requested that Prime Minister Diefenbaker establish a Royal Commission on healthcare. They fully expected this committee to make recommendations in line with the private, fee-for-service insurance model they were proposing. Diefenbaker quickly acquiesced to their request and established a seven-member *Royal Commission on Health Services*, under the leadership of Justice Emmett Hall.

This commission's mandate was to:

> *"Inquire into and report upon the existing facilities and the future needs for health services for the people of Canada and the resources to provide such services, and to recommend such measures, consistent with the constitutional division of legislative powers in Canada, as commissioners believe will ensure that the best possible healthcare is available to all Canadians."[102]*

The commission was comprised of a surgeon, a dentist, and a former president of the Saskatchewan Medical Association—a committee membership that, at first glance, appeared favorable to the CMA's position. Hall himself was a Saskatchewan Supreme Court justice, who was elevated to the Canadian Supreme Court in 1962. His personal views were unknown, but he had run for office in the provincial legislature against the CCF in 1948, suggesting that he was opposed to many of their policies.

Led by Hall, the Royal Commission on Health Services reviewed 406 Briefs and 26 research reports, and listened to 67 days of public hearings in all provinces and the Yukon territories. The commission took three years to generate its report, which was first released in the House of Commons on June 19, 1964—with a final version issued on December 7, 1964.

The report unanimously recommended a national health policy that was modeled on the Saskatchewan Medicare program, stating:

> *"Health services must not be denied to certain individuals simply because the latter make no contribution to the economic development of Canada or because he cannot pay for such*

---

[102]   Health Canada website: Royal Commission on Health Services, 1961-1964: http://www.hc-sc.gc.ca/hcs-sss/com/fed/hall-eng.php (accessed May 23rd, 2015)

services. Important as economics is, we must also take into account the human and spiritual aspects involved."[103]

Progressive Conservative Prime Minister John Diefenbaker had requested the Royal Commission on Health Services report. When the report was delivered in 1964, the Liberals under Prime Minister Lester Pearson had resumed power. He and his party were under no obligation to act upon this report. However, they recognized the benefits it outlined and realized the public support for this initiative. Slowly, they worked to put the recommendations in place.

Despite the resistance of Canadian physicians, the *Medical Care Act of Canada* (commonly known as the *Medicare Act*) became law in 1966 and took effect on July 1, 1968.[104] The *Medicare Act* outlined the manner in which universal, public coverage of hospital and physician services would be provided to all Canadians. It did not address funding of other critical aspects of healthcare, such as the cost of prescription medications and long-term care (LTC) facilities.

When the *Medicare Act* was passed into law by a vote of 177 to 2 in 1966, it ensured that physician services for the sick and injured would be publicly funded—pending provincial approval. This, combined with the *HIDS Act* of 1957, meant that the two major elements of healthcare provision of the day (physician services and hospital care) were now fully funded by the government.

However, at its core, Medicare was a means to fund these elements of healthcare—not an approach to how healthcare itself should be organized and delivered. Ironically and tragically, the nature of the funding mechanism—separate payments for hospital services and physician services—effectively served to lock in a system of healthcare delivery, which now all but guarantees poorly-coordinated, fragmented care. This approach has grown increasingly dysfunctional as the nature of healthcare delivery has evolved.

---

[103] Vaughan, Fredrick. *Aggressive in Pursuit: The Life of Justice Emmett Hall.* p. 128. Osgoode Society for Canadian Legal History, 2004.

[104] http://www.historymuseum.ca/cmc/exhibitions/hist/medicare/medic-5h24e.shtml

As part of the *Medicare Act*, the federal government committed to providing matching funding to the provinces for hospital care and physician services. In turn, each province was responsible for how that care was organized and delivered. By specifically funding only care that was delivered via hospitals, it made sense for provincial governments to promote these entities. Soon, most healthcare funding flowed through large hospital entities. Similarly, by funding individual physician services on a fee-for-service basis, an individual-oriented, physician-centric approach to care delivery became the norm. This funding structure created, and then subsequently reinforced, a now archaic care delivery model.

Canadian Healthcare from Medicare to the Canada Health Act (1968-1984)

In April of 1972, the Yukon territories ratified the Medicare agreement, signifying that all provinces and territories within Canada had now approved the *Medical Care Act*. Canada now had universal healthcare. However, even before this date, some problematic issues related to public funding of healthcare had become plainly manifest.

The costs of funding this system proved to be much larger than expected. Healthcare costs were increasing at 15% a year in 1975, and 16% a year by 1980. This, combined with the marked economic downturn of the 1970s, led to rapidly increasing budget deficits at both the federal and provincial levels. This, in turn, led to tense arguments over how the funding would continue. Additionally, many noted that Canadians were not getting the healthcare system they had expected. A number of physicians were still "extra billing"—charging patients more than the negotiated rates. Furthermore, there were early signs that the healthcare being delivered was not what would be expected, given the extensive outlay of funds.

The *Medical Care Act* established that the federal government would fund 50% of both hospital services and physician services. However, as these costs rose dramatically, the federal government became increasingly frustrated that they were stuck with such a large bill, yet had no real oversight on how the provincial governments spent the money. There was a growing concern that the provinces were siphoning off some of the federal funding—and using this for budgets not related to healthcare. In 1976, the liberal government under Prime Minister Pierre Trudeau decided, without the provinces' consent, to place limits on the growth rate of their financial transfer payments. Needless to say, this frustrated and angered their provincial counterparts.

Intense arguments also ensued between the physicians and the provincial and federal governments. During the early years of Medicare, many physicians did very well financially. Many changed the way they organized and ran their practices. The provincially-negotiated rates physicians now charged were much lower than they had previously charged. However, every patient now had insurance, so by seeing more patients, physicians were able to recoup any lost income. Furthermore, many physicians had previously seen uninsured or underinsured patients for little or no compensation. Now this group of patients had full insurance, creating a new, and often lucrative, revenue source. The cost of funding physician services soared. In many ways, this was the golden era of physician remuneration in Canada.

Subsequently, provincial governments began to tighten up the rules on physician funding, making it more difficult for physicians to reach what they believed was a satisfactory income level. The physicians' response to this was to rely, in many instances, on user fees or balanced billing— essentially charging patients the difference between what the provincial governments were paying them for each service rendered and the fees their Provincial Medical Associations had established. This infuriated those running the health system at the federal and provincial levels.

With the escalating disagreement in funding between the provincial and federal governments, as well as the conflict between the physicians and the governments, it was time for another commission. In June of 1979, the Progressive Conservatives, under the leadership of Joe Clark, defeated Pierre Trudeau's liberals and established a minority government. The health minister, David Crombie, like Monique Begin, his Liberal predecessor, came under increasing pressure to resolve these feuds. In September of 1979, Crombie called for another report on the healthcare system, albeit with less resources and a tighter timeline than the 1964 commission.

Emmett Hall, now 81 years old, was again chosen to write this report. He was given a broad mandate.[105] However, two clear issues were front and center: Were the provincial governments using their federal health transfer funding appropriately? And did user fees and extra billing by hospitals and physicians undermine the goals of Medicare?

Once again, Hall travelled across the country, listening to citizens, medical groups, and the provincial government representatives. In addition, he reviewed 450 briefs from various individuals and groups, related to the healthcare system. His report, *Canada's National-Provincial Health Program for the 1980s: A Commitment for Renewal*, was published on August 29th, 1980.[106] The report reaffirmed the essential elements of universal healthcare in Canada. It refuted the federal government's claim that the provinces had been inappropriately using the federal transfer payments to fund non-healthcare services. However, it strongly criticized user fees and extra billing, claiming that they undermined the principles of universal medical care. This second Hall report eventually became the foundation for the 1984 *Canada Health Act*.

On March 3, 1980, the Federal Liberals, led by Pierre Trudeau, returned to power with a majority government. Prime Minister Trudeau again appointed Monique Begin as Health Minister. Physicians

---

[105]   http://www.hc-sc.gc.ca/hcs-sss/com/fed/hs-ss-79-eng.php
Mandate for the 1979 Hall report:
-Report on progress made on national health policy since the Royal commission in 1964
-Examine the extent to which principles of portability, reasonable access, universal coverage, comprehensive coverage, public administration, and uniform terms and conditions were being achieved
-Consider whether there should be other basic principles for health insurance delivery
-Consider the nature and extent of necessary revisions to the Hospital Insurance and Diagnostic Services Act, the Medical Care Act, and related legislation
-Consider other ways public authorities could comply with principles in the act

[106]   *Canada's National-Provincial Health Program for the 1980's: A Commitment for Renewal.* http://www.hc-sc.gc.ca/hcs-sss/com/fed/hs-ss-79-eng.php (Accessed December 6th 2015)

naturally opposed any restriction on their billing practices. Many of the provincial governments had sided with the physicians, as a means to appease them. Therefore, they also supported, or at least accepted, extra billing. Resistance by these powerful groups was countered by public sentiment.

Going directly to the people and over the heads of physician groups and the provincial governments, Monique Begin held many public forums in 1982. Based on the feedback she received, the governing federal Liberal party became convinced that they represented the will of the people. Despite resistance from provincial governments and outright hostility from physician groups, the principles outlined in Emmett Hall's 1980 report evolved into the *Canada Health Act*, which was passed by the federal legislature and received Royal Assent on April 1, 1984.

At its core, the *Canada Health Act* is about funding healthcare. It outlines the criteria that must be met in order for provincial governments to receive federal healthcare transfer payments. It does *not* provide any specific details about how healthcare should be organized and practiced, just the criteria that must be met in order for provinces to receive funding. Furthermore, the funding question applies only to hospital services and physician services. Many healthcare services, representing approximately 30% of the healthcare dollars spent in Canada, fall outside of the jurisdiction of the *Canada Health Act*. This includes critically important healthcare areas such as prescription medications and long-term care (LTC) costs.

The primary objective of the *Canada Health Act*, as listed in the preamble, is:

> *To protect, promote and restore the physical and mental wellbeing of residents of Canada and to facilitate reasonable access to health services without financial or other barriers.* [107]
> It lays out five conditions that must be met, in order for provinces to receive federal transfer payments. These criteria are:

---

[107]   Canada Health Act. R.S.C. 1985, c. C-6. P. 5. (http://laws-lois.justice.gc.ca/ PDF/C-6.pdf Accessed April 24th, 2015)

1. Public administration
2. Comprehensiveness
3. Universality
4. Portability
5. Accessibility

The **public administration** criterion ensures that the healthcare system will be run, directly or indirectly, by the provincial governments. It states: "Administered and operated on a nonprofit basis by a public authority, responsible to the provincial/territorial governments and subject to audits of their accounts and financial transactions." This provision recognizes that healthcare funding is a de facto insurance, and this criterion prevents for-profit insurance companies from being involved in administering the public healthcare system. However, it does NOT prevent provincial governments from delegating care delivery and management to other entities.

The **comprehensiveness** provision states that: "All insured health services provided by hospitals, medical practitioners or dentists" must be covered by the public health plan. Dental services are only covered if they are performed within a hospital setting. This distinction is based on earlier definitions about which care would be covered. The provinces have the option of extending coverage to other areas (e.g., dentists and midwives), but for financial reasons, they often do not do this.

The **universality** criterion establishes that all insured persons would be eligible for health services, "provided for by the plan on uniform terms and conditions." This section ensures that once an individual is designated as an insured person, he or she will be eligible for all aspects of healthcare insurance. There are exceptions to this criterion, such as individuals working within the Armed Forces, inmates at federal penitentiaries, individuals covered under the provincial Worker's Compensation laws, and some aboriginal groups.

The **portability** criterion was established to ensure that Canadians would be free to travel and move about the country without concerns regarding their healthcare coverage. This criterion establishes the need for each provincial healthcare system to accept and provide coverage to citizens from other provinces.

The fifth criterion, **accessibility**, may be the most controversial. This criteria states that the insurance plan must provide for "reasonable access," and that this access must be "on uniform terms and conditions, unprecluded, unimpeded, either directly or indirectly, by charges (user charges or extra billing) or other means (age, health status or financial circumstances)." Although this section also provided for "reasonable compensation" for healthcare providers, physicians across the country vehemently opposed this element of the *Canada Health Act*. The "accessibility" provision effectively banned extra billing and forced provincial governments to stop this practice—if they wished to continue receiving federal funds. The provincial governments had no choice but to comply.

From the Canada Health Act to the Romanow Report (1985-2002)

With the passage of the *Canada Health Act*, all provinces now needed to work toward banning extra billing by physicians. This mandate would run headlong into the physicians' adamant refusal to have their fees controlled entirely by each provincial government. On December 20, 1985, the Ontario government introduced the *Healthcare Accessibility Act*, which effectively banned extra billing. After a failure to negotiate a satisfactory agreement between the province and the doctors, a series of physician office closures were carried out in May of 1986.[108]

Finally, on June 12, 1986, the doctors of Ontario, with support from the Ontario Medical Association and the Canadian Medical Association, went on strike. Many, but not all, physicians stopped providing care. A number of emergency rooms in the Toronto area closed. The withdrawal of physician services became so widespread that the College of Physicians and Surgeons of Ontario intervened, formally reminding physicians of their obligation to provide essential services—lest they face charges for professional misconduct.

Throughout the strike, the public remained steadfast in its support of the provincial governments. They did not see the physicians' concerns as valid. After 25 days, the doctors were broken—they capitulated to the

---

[108] http://www.historymuseum.ca/cmc/exhibitions/hist/medicare/medic-7h11e. shtml

Ontario government's demands and the strike ended. The ban on extra billing dictated by the *Canada Health Act* was here to stay. With this ban came tighter oversight of compensation that physicians could receive. However, the bill did nothing to change the fact that physicians were still viewed as independent businesspeople, free to run their practice as they saw fit—with respect to the patients they saw and the procedures they performed.

In the early 1990s, the Medicare Act, which ensured government funding of physician services, had been in place for a quarter of a century—and the *Hospital Insurance and Diagnostic Service Act* (HIDS Act) for 35 years. Canadians had come to enjoy the concept of universal health coverage and revered their idealized view of the public health system. However, this was not a time for celebration. The largely unseen expenses associated with providing public healthcare was staggering and continuing to grow. Furthermore, because healthcare was not a system, but rather a means for funding physician and hospital care, there was no easy way to rein in cost growth and simultaneously improve healthcare quality.

When I graduated from McGill medical school in 1991, a few of my classmates started a two-year, family medicine residency program, while the vast majority of us headed off to do a year of rotating internship. After this, many started working as General Practitioners (GPs), while the rest of us began residency training in our specialty of choice. Within three years, that had all changed. By the mid 1990s, medical schools had cut admissions by an average of 5.9%, the rotating internship had been eliminated, and GPs were on a path to eventual extinction—being replaced by residency trained family practice physicians.[109]

The main reason for these changes came down to finances. Doctors are expensive—not just in the pay they receive, but in the expenses they generate within the system. In the early 1990s many Canadian healthcare experts predicted an oversupply of physicians.[110] For a healthcare system reeling from costs that were increasing much

---

[109] Evans RG, MacGrail KM. Richard III, Barer-Stoddard and the Daughter of Time. Healthcare Policy Vol 3 No 3, 2008.

[110] Primary Care Physicians: Managing Supply in Canada, Germany, Sweden, and the United Kingdom (Letter Report, 05/18/94, GAO/HEHS-94-111).

faster than inflation, decreasing one of the main cost drivers must have seemed like a good idea.

The proposal to decrease the physician supply in Canada as a means to help control healthcare costs is attributed to the Barer-Stoddart report.[111] This report was commissioned for the 1991 Federal/Provincial/Territorial Conference of Deputy Ministers of Health. The authors, Morris Barer and Greg Stoddart, were both highly-respected academics. The report outlined 53 recommendations that aimed to decrease healthcare costs and improve performance. The authors warned that "cherry picking" would undermine the integrated nature of the recommendations and potentially do more harm than good.[26] Despite this, only three of their recommendations were implemented: decreasing medical school admissions by 10%, reducing the number of residency positions, and decreasing the reliance on foreign trained doctors.[112]

The health ministries focused on implementing these three recommendations and began cutting the supply of physicians beginning in the mid-1990s. Unfortunately, they ignored most of the other recommendations, including the suggestion to increase coordination of healthcare provision—and other recommendations designed to create a more integrated, coordinated healthcare system. Combined with a greater-than-expected loss of practicing physicians in Canada, the absence of a move to meaningfully redesign the system, as suggested by the Barer-Stoddart report and others, led to substantial problems by the end of the decade.

Throughout the 1990s many physician became increasingly frustrated with the Canadian medical system due to issues related to compensation and practice satisfaction. This combined with limited

---

[111] Barer ML, Stoddart CL. *Toward integrated medical resource policies for Canada*. Prepared for the Federal/Provincial/Territorial Conference of Deputy Ministers of Health. Winnipeg: Conference of Deputy Ministers of Health, Manitoba Health; June 1991. Published in a 12-part series in CMAJ1992;146(3) to 1993;148(1).

[112] Nadeem Esmail. Southern Border Without Doctors: Canada's failed efforts at central planning have created a physician shortage. *National Review Online*, Sept 6th 2006. http://www.freerepublic.com/focus/f-news/1696628/posts (accessed December 7th 2015)

job opportunity for newly trained graduates caused many physicians to move to the United States. In 1996 there was a net loss of 513 physicians leaving Canada, the equivalent of 30% of the annual output from Canada's 16 medical schools.[113] The immigration of physicians to the United States combined with smaller numbers of medical school graduates, more physicians in longer, specialty residency training programs, and a purported increase in middle-aged physicians who decided to retire led to a noticeable decrease in available physician services by the end of the decade.

By the year 2000, the problem governments faced was not so much a lack of physicians; excellent care could have been rendered with the available physicians, had it been coordinated and integrated. Rather, the "problem" for governments was the perceived shortage of Canadian physicians. This resulted in a dramatic increase in the power of the Canadian Medical Association and the provincial medical associations, who now found themselves in a strong bargaining position when negotiating with their Ministry of Health counterparts.

Increasing dissatisfaction with access and care that patients received within the public system led to an increase in private medicine, beginning in the mid 1990s. The *Canada Health Act* had created the impetus for provinces to ban extra billing. Physicians stopped this practice but still found numerous creative ways to essentially function within a private system. Various private clinics, concierge practices, and even private surgery centers began to appear.

Perhaps the most well known was the Vancouver-based Cambie Surgery Center, founded in 1996 by Dr. Brian Day—one of the attending orthopaedic surgeons at my residency training program. Despite private pay surgery being technically illegal under the guidelines set forth by the *Canada Health Act*, this and other surgery centers have prospered, due to enough demand for expedited surgical care. Often, their biggest clients have been the provincial governments themselves, via the province-run Worker's Compensation programs—specifically because it is so prohibitively expensive to pay injured workers while they wait months for surgery.

---

[113]   Gray C. How bad is the brain drain? CMAJ 1999;161:1028-9

Canadian Healthcare Since the Romanow Report (2002-Present)

The perceived doctor shortage, increasing private healthcare, and healthcare costs that continued to rise much faster than inflation created the impetus for another royal commission on healthcare in 2001. On the recommendation of Prime Minister Jean Chrétien's federal government, the mandate for this commission stated:

> *"Inquire into and undertake dialogue with Canadians on the future of Canada's public health care system, and to recommend policies and measures respectful of the jurisdictions and powers in Canada required to ensure over the long term the sustainability of a universally accessible, publicly funded health system that offers quality services to Canadians and strikes an appropriate balance between investments in prevention and health maintenance and those directed to care and treatment."[114]*

The federal government led by Prime Minister Jean Chrétien asked Roy Romanow, former Premier of Manitoba, to lead the commission. He began by reviewing the facts of the existing system, and then moved to a public dialogue with Canadians. On November 28, 2002, he presented his report, *Building on Values: The Future of Health Care in Canada*, to the House of Commons.

The Romanow report presents a comprehensive review of the existing healthcare system that passionately reinforced the value and importance of the publically funded healthcare system. However, a major flaw has undermined its ultimate effectiveness. The report made 47 specific recommendations. The first was a recommitment to a "universally accessible, publicly funded health care system" -or at least the hospital and physician component of this system established by *HIDS* and the *Medicare Act*. Other recommendations included increased federal funding of healthcare via a Canada Health Transfer, an increased focus on electronic health records to facilitate improved care, a fundamental reform of the manner in which aboriginal healthcare was managed and administered, and a focus on performance metrics and outcomes to assess and ensure accountability of the existing health system.

---

[114] Minutes from a meeting of the Privy Council on April 3, 2001 (P.C. 2001-569).

The recommendations from the Romanow report were well reasoned, and many were subsequently incorporated into public policy. For example, the federal government introduced the *Canada Health and Social Transfer Program* on April 1, 2004. Subsequently, health transfer payments from the federal government to the provinces increased by an average of 6% per year for a decade. This noticeable increase in federal funding of healthcare has allowed the Canadian government to make healthcare responsibility primarily a political issue for the provinces—by removing the persistent complaint that they were not adequately funding the system.

In hindsight, the most profound flaw of the Romanow report was that it did not recommend fundamental system reorganization, although the report did recognize this problem:

> *"We also need to renovate our concept of Medicare and adapt it to today's realities. In the early days, Medicare could be summarized in two words: hospitals and doctors. That was fine for the time, but it is not sufficient for the 21ˢᵗ century. Despite the tremendous changes over the past 40 years, Medicare still is largely organized around hospitals and doctors."[115]*

However, the Romanow report did not then outline any meaningful change to address the structural organization of the health system that propagated this approach to healthcare delivery. It did not seem to fully appreciate that the heart of the matter was the existing manner in which care was delivered; hospitals receive bulk funding, regardless of performance, with care provided by isolated physicians paid on a fee-for-service basis.

A senate report written by Michael Kirby issued immediately after the Romanow report in December 2002 identified this problem:

> *"First, our report proposes that the way in which hospitals are funded be transformed. We believe we must move away from the current practice of giving hospitals global budgets based largely on historical spending patterns. Instead, we propose to fund hospitals on the basis of the services that they*

---

[115] *Building on Values: The Future of Health Care in Canada*, p. xvii. Commissioner: Roy J. Romanow, Q.C., November 2002.

actually deliver. Many of these difficulties can be traced to a misalignment of incentives with desired behaviour. Fee-for-service remuneration rewards episodic more than continuing care, fast 'through-put' of patients, and dealing with simple procedures more than challenging ones."[116]

Therefore, while the Romanow report led to changes, such as increased federal funding and an increased emphasis on outcome metrics, it did not fundamentally alter the way care was funded and subsequently delivered. The Canadian healthcare system limped forward.

Today, many Canadians still love their healthcare system, or at least their concept of what they want their healthcare system to be: public, universal, and comprehensive. However, there is increasing evidence that Canadians are recognizing that they are not getting good value from their healthcare system. Financially, healthcare costs have become the elephant in the room for all provincial finance ministers. From a care delivery point of view, evidence is increasingly echoing my experience: Canadian healthcare is expensive and inefficient, and it delivers care that is on the whole mediocre—or worse.[117]

Summary: Chapter 5

Today, the NHL is synonymous with professional hockey, and it is always looking to do what is in the best interest of the NHL. Individual NHL teams still battle ferociously against each other, but they do so within a set of rules and an organizing structure that is designed to better the league as a whole. Team owners realize that if the league does well, they will do well. Similarly, players realize that what is in their own best interests is, invariably, to be the best team player they can be for their team.

---

[116]   Response to the Romanow Report. Standing Senate Committee on Social Affairs, Science and Technology. Chair: Michael Kirby, December 2002. http://www.parl.gc.ca/content/sen/committee/372/soci/press/04dec02-e.htm

[117]   The Commonwealth Fund: *Mirror, Mirror on the Wall, 2014 Update: How the U.S. Health Care System Compares Internationally.* Karen Davis, Kristof Stremikis, David Squires, Cathy Schoen. Published June 16th 2014: http://www.commonwealthfund.org/publications/fund-reports/2014/jun/mirror-mirror

This is a far cry from hockey prior to 1925—when professional leagues battled against other leagues, owners argued with other owners, and the game itself often emphasized the performance of individual players over team play (as illustrated by the lack of emphasis on passing). In many ways, the Canadian healthcare system is akin to professional hockey prior to 1925. The rules of play have not been appropriately updated, individual players (i.e., doctors) are emphasized over team play, and there is little to no meaningful coordination between teams (i.e., hospitals and other venues for healthcare delivery) within the league (i.e., the health ministries).

Professional hockey had a major, disruptive upheaval in the years leading up to 1925. During that time, rules were fundamentally changed to improve the game, followed by a steady evolution—in order to constantly enhance the game and increase its appeal to fans. Canadian healthcare needs to change the rules by which it is organized, but it has not been able to do this because of outdated rules that have become ensconced in the existing healthcare system.

What this chapter has attempted to illustrate is that history has played a huge part—and at times, an unfortunate role—in how Canadian healthcare is delivered today. Healthcare is a provincial jurisdiction today because "healthcare" in 1867, at the time of confederation, was considered sanitation management—something that needed to be coordinated locally—not disease management, for which there were no consistent cures back then. Healthcare is funded and delivered largely through a hospital-based organizational structure today, despite other much more effective and efficient delivery methods, because of a federal healthcare funding law that was passed in 1957 and persists today.

Physicians cannot easily be brought into a team-based structure that is the essence of today's healthcare system because they are still largely treated as private businesspeople, who are paid on a fee-for-service basis—just as they were compensated in 1966 when the *Medicare Act* passed. Understanding history gives us a chance to more effectively create a new pathway forward. In the final chapters of this book, I will argue that this pathway should be based on established principles of effective, modern healthcare delivery.

Summary Points: Chapter 5

The present-day Canadian healthcare system owes much of its structure to the quirks of history.

Healthcare in Canada is a provincial jurisdiction by designation of the *British North America Act of 1867* because in that era, healthcare primarily involved ensuring appropriate local sanitation.

In the 1800s hospitals were largely for the poor and destitute with middle- and upper-class Canadians typically receiving medical care in their homes or at their personal physician's office. By the 1950s, the development of sophisticated diagnostic equipment, improved treatments, and increased surgical success established hospitals as the primary place for patients to receive care for serious medical issues.

The *Hospital Insurance and Diagnostic Services (HIDS) Act* of 1957 guaranteed the federal government would match provincial funding for the costs of hospital-related services.

The federal *Medicare Act* came into effect in 1968. This act established that all physician services would now be covered by each provincial government with matching federal funding. This combined with the HIDS Act ensured universal healthcare for all Canadians—at least for physicians' services and hospital-related care.

The *Canada Health Act* of 1984 clarified the criteria that must be met for provincial governments to receive federal funding for healthcare but did not address how healthcare should be organized and delivered.

CHAPTER 6

A Primer on 21st Century Healthcare Delivery

Walter: *It's a tough draw even if we don't play the Soviets. What the hell happens if we do?*

Lou Nanne: *We put our best on the ice with them last year. Professional all-stars. They still beat us.*

Herb Brooks: *It wasn't because you weren't good enough... All-star teams fail because they rely solely on the individual's talent. The Soviets win because they take that talent and use it inside a system that's designed for the betterment of the team.*

*From the movie **Miracle** (Disney 2004)—The story of the United States hockey team's victory over the powerhouse Soviet Union in the 1980 Olympic Games.*

Introduction

Being an orthopaedic resident at a children's hospital is busy, but it is also usually enjoyable. Most kids are joyful and innocent, even when they are sick or injured. Furthermore, the type of people who choose to work with children tend to go out of their way to create a happy, caring, and positive environment. Ward 3C at the large children's hospital I trained at epitomized this attitude. It was where the orthopaedic patients were admitted, a space we shared with other surgical disciplines and some of the oncology patients. The ward was a beehive of activity, with high-energy, caring, happy staff interacting with the myriad of children admitted to the ward.

However, late one October morning in 1995, that was not the case when I visited the ward to assess one of the orthopaedic patients between surgeries. No one on the ward seemed to be moving. There was an eerie silence, broken only by the uncontrolled sobbing of one of the middle-aged nurses. I quietly approached the long-time unit clerk and, in a whisper, asked, "What happened?" Looking down, she whispered back, "One of the oncology patients just received an intrathecal injection of chemotherapy that was supposed to be given intravenously."

This was bad... Very bad! Chemotherapeutic agents such as cisplatinum kill rapidly-growing cells when injected into the bloodstream, but when injected into the spinal fluid, the medication wreaks havoc on the spinal cord and brain. The patient, a 12-year-old girl who was in remission from leukemia, was raced off to the operating room in a heroic—but ultimately futile—attempt to flush the chemotherapeutic agents from her spinal fluid. She died a week later. The chemotherapy she had received up till that point had essentially cured her of her cancer. She was killed by the medical system.

As medicine moved toward the end of the 20th century, it became apparent to those observing healthcare systems that these types of medical errors were ubiquitous. The mistakes themselves were not necessarily common. However, the system was treating so many patients that even something that occurred in one out of 1,000—or even one out of 100,000—times would end up happening quite often. X-rays and lab tests were ordered and then not checked for the results. Medication errors occurred—either the wrong dose or the wrong medication was prescribed, or it was administered incorrectly, as with the patient above. Surgery was performed on the wrong extremity, the wrong operation was performed on the wrong patient, or the wrong type of blood was transfused into a patient. These types of errors, and many others, were now happening with frightening regularity at almost all hospitals.

These types of mistakes were not mistakes due to lack of knowledge or skill, nor were they a product of an uncaring doctor or nurse. The oncology fellow who administered the fatal intrathecal injection at the children's hospital knew certain drugs should never be injected into the spinal canal. She simply made a mistake—a mistake that killed the patient, devastated the patient's family, and likely shattered her own career.

Perhaps the package the medication came in looked very similar to medication that is injected into the spinal canal. Perhaps the oncology fellow was exhausted from being up all night on call. Perhaps she was overwhelmed with work and rushing to catch up. Regardless of the reason, she did what humans do—she made a mistake. Systems need to be designed with this fact in mind.

In most instances, medical errors cannot be definitively attributed to a single individual. Usually they occur from a combination of events. They occur because human beings make mistakes. They occur because the traditional healthcare system was not designed in a way that protects patients from these mistakes—and the various other ways that medical errors occurred.

To Err is Human

By the 1990s, there was a growing realization that no amount of memorizing of facts by medical students, yelling or screaming at residents during their training, or intense basic science research, was going to eliminate these types of medical errors. A different approach was required—an approach that addressed the medical system, not the individuals working within the system.

In 1998, the *Institute of Medicine* (IOM) formed the Committee on Quality of Health Care in America. This committee was charged with "developing a strategy that would result in substantial improvement in the quality of health care over the next 10 years."[118] Their first report, based on a detailed literature review, examined medical errors. The resulting landmark report, *To Err is Human: Building a Safer Health System*, was published in 1999.

The IOM was founded in 1970 under the jurisdiction of the United States' National Academy of Sciences. It is a nonprofit, nongovernmental organization, committed to providing "unbiased authoritative advice to decision-makers and the public" on issues related to medicine and healthcare.[119] While many of the reports are generated at the request of the United States Congress, the organization is committed to providing independent guidance that is based on the available literature.

Membership in the IOM is a prestigious honor. Healthcare professionals are nominated and elected by existing members of the IOM, based on distinguished contributions and service to medicine. Election to the IOM is not only an honor, it is also a commitment to provide service to improve medicine and the healthcare system. While not a Canadian organization, the IOM is committed to accurately reflecting the worldwide scientific literature. Canadian medical schools and residency trainings are under similar jurisdictions as their American counterparts, and hospitals have been organized and accredited in similar manners. As such, findings of the IOM are directly applicable to the Canadian healthcare system.

One of the central conclusions of *To Err is Human: Building a Safer Health System* was that medical errors caused between 44,000 and 98,000 unnecessary deaths each year in US hospitals. This represents between 2-4% of all deaths in the United States. When *To Err is Human* was released, physicians, healthcare workers, and the general public were incredulous about these figures. However, over time there have been reluctant realizations that not only are these results probably accurate, they may underrepresent the problem.

---

[118] *To Err is Human: Building a Safer Medical System*. Institute of Medicine. P. 1, November 1999.

[119] Institute of Medicine. Advising the Nation/Improving Health (https://www.nationalacademies.org/hmd/~/media/Files/About%20the%20IOM/IOM-brochure-website.pdf Accessed July 2nd 2016)

The figures themselves were generated by extrapolating from two major research studies.[120,121] One study was based on data from Colorado and Utah that found medical errors occurred in 2.9% of patients who had been hospitalized. This was compared to a 3.7% adverse-event rate among hospitalized patients in a large study of New York hospitals. More detailed analysis of these errors demonstrated that, in the Colorado and Utah study, the errors led to patient death in 6.6% of patients, whereas in the New York study, they led to death in 13.6% of patients. Extrapolating these results over the entire population of hospitalized patients in the United States led to the conclusion that death related to medical error was between 44,000 and 98,000 patients each year.

To Err is Human was clear to point out that medical errors were often *system errors*—the products of "the decentralized and fragmented nature of the healthcare delivery system."[122] As such, they stated, "The focus must shift from blaming individuals for past errors to focus on preventing future errors by designing safety into the system."[123]

The report identified two types of errors:

1. Errors of execution: The correct action does not proceed as intended.
2. Errors of planning: The original, intended action is not correct.

The report presented a number of recommendations, including delineating the ultimate target of all the recommendations, which was intended to create safety systems inside healthcare organizations

---

[120]   Brennan TA, Leape LL, Laird NM, Hebert L, Localio AR, Lawthers AG, Newhouse JP, Weiler PC, Hiatt HH. Incidence of adverse events and negligence in hospitalized patients. Results of the Harvard Medical Practice Study I. *N Engl J Med*. 1991 Feb 7;324(6):370-6

[121]   Thomas EJ, Studdert DM, Burstin HR, Orav EJ, Zeena T, Williams EJ, Howard KM, Weiler PC, Brennan TA. Incidence and types of adverse events and negligent care in Utah and Colorado. *Med Care*. 200 Mar;38(3):261-71

[122]   *To Err is Human: Building a Safer Medical System*. Institute of Medicine. P. 3, November 1999.

[123]   *To Err is Human: Building a Safer Medical System*. Institute of Medicine. P. 5, November 1999.

through the implementation of safe practices at the delivery level.[124] In addition, they emphasized using the experience of other "high-risk industries" to improve healthcare safety.[125] The enduring legacy of *To Err is Human* has been the realization that healthcare delivery could no longer be business as usual.

Crossing the Quality Chasm

In 2001, the IOM published *Crossing the Quality Chasm: A New Health System for the 21st Century*. This was the second and final report of the IOM's Committee on Quality of Health Care in America. It was released in 2001, a little more than a year after *To Err is Human*. However, whereas *To Err is Human* focused specifically on the epidemic of medical errors, *Crossing the Quality Chasm* looked at the entire healthcare system as it pertained to quality and safety. The conclusion of the report was unequivocal; fundamental reform of healthcare was needed:

> *"The current care system cannot do the job. Trying harder will not work. Changing systems of care will."*[126]

Crossing the Quality Chasm pointed out that there was a fragmented nature of care in traditional healthcare systems, and that physician groups, hospitals, and other healthcare organizations operate as silos. In other words, different hospital departments and organizations were functioning in isolation from each other. This report was a clear call for action to improve the American healthcare delivery system as a whole. The report itself was not prescriptive. Rather, it laid out specific aims and goals that the system should aspire to. It defined what the end result should look like in general terms. Additionally, it identified

---

[124] *To Err is Human: Building a Safer Medical System*. Institute of Medicine. P. 6, November 1999.

[125] *To Err is Human: Building a Safer Medical System*. Institute of Medicine. P. 13, November 1999.

[126] *Crossing the Quality Chasm: A New Health System for the 21st Century*. A report of the *Institute of Medicine's* Committee on Quality of Health Care in America. P.4, 2001.

a series of principles that the health systems should follow in order to achieve these gains.

Crossing the Quality Chasm sent a message to the medical world that the existing way of practicing medicine was falling far short of its potential. It confirmed a suspicion that many physicians, healthcare practitioners, administrators, and patients had harboured for a number of years. It did not give specific answers to how this problem should be solved. However, it also made it clear that the solution to what ailed the healthcare system would not be found merely by tinkering around the edges. Fundamental system redesign would be necessary.

One of the primary things that *Crossing the Quality Chasm* did was outline what the aims of a good healthcare system should be. The report stated that those providing healthcare should work to "continually reduce the burden of illness, injury, and disability, and to improve the health and functioning of the people of the United States."[127] They went further in their second recommendation, defining six aims for healthcare. They stated that it should be safe, effective, patient-centred, timely, efficient, and equitable (see Table 2).

With respect to how a healthcare organization achieves these aims, they were not specific. However, they did outline a series of basic rules to guide healthcare reform.[128] These rules emphasized the importance of the patient's perspective and the need to have a coordinated, integrated, and cooperative healthcare team that is designed to consistently achieve the desired end result of care. They specifically emphasized the importance of the system over individual actors within the system. In addition, they emphasized evidence-based, rather than idiosyncratic, decision-making, as well as the need for continuous quality-improvement processes.

---

[127] *Crossing the Quality Chasm: A New Health System for the 21ˢᵗ Century.* A report of the *Institute of Medicine's* Committee on Quality of Health Care in America. P.39, 2001

[128] *Crossing the Quality Chasm: A New Health System for the 21ˢᵗ Century.* A report of the *Institute of Medicine's* Committee on Quality of Health Care in America. Chapter 3: Formulating New Rules to Redesign and Improve Care. P. 61-88, 2001.

Table 2: Six Specific Aims for Improving Healthcare[129]

Healthcare should be:

1. **Safe**: avoiding injuries to patients from the care that is intended to help them
2. **Effective**: providing services, based on scientific knowledge to all who could benefit, and refraining from providing services to those not likely to benefit (i.e., avoiding underuse and overuse)
3. **Patient-centred**: providing care that is respectful of, and responsive to, individual patient preferences, needs, and values, and ensuring that patient values guide all clinical decisions
4. **Timely**: reducing wait times and (sometimes) harmful delays, for both those who receive and those who give care
5. **Efficient**: avoiding waste, in particular waste of equipment, supplies, ideas, and energy
6. **Equitable**: providing care that does not vary in quality because of personal characteristics, such as gender, ethnicity, geographic location, and socioeconomic status

The rules they outlined would likely seem logical and self-evident to an outside observer—healthcare as a team event, working to address each patient's goals in a systematic manner. However, they were very different from the practical reality of what was happening within most existing healthcare systems.

Both seminal reports from the Institute of Medicine were American in origin. However, the ideas contained in these reports had universal applicability. Good healthcare does not have geographical or ideological borders. These ideas served as a powerful wake-up call that fundamental change was needed—change that was predicated on system redesign.

---

[129] *Crossing the Quality Chasm: A New Health System for the 21st Century*. A report of the *Institute of Medicine's* Committee on Quality of Health Care in America. P.39-40, 2001

The Triple Aim: A Population-Based, Diabetic Foot Program

58-year-old Janice Smith, who had long-standing diabetes, presented to our emergency room one April with a deep, foul-smelling ulcer on her right foot. The decreased sensation, poor circulation, and compromised healing capacity that resulted from her chronic diabetes had all contributed to a sequence of events that led to the development of her serious foot infection. She needed to be admitted to the hospital and aggressively treated.

An animated argument ensued between the orthopaedic service and the vascular service over who would have to admit this patient and thereby lose one of their precious hospital beds.[130] In this instance, orthopaedics lost the argument, and she was admitted to our service. Janice underwent three operations over the next 10 days in an effort to eradicate the infection from her foot. She was discharged only to return to the emergency room three weeks later. The infection had reoccurred, and the only option was to amputate her lower leg.

Serious diabetic foot infections, like the one that claimed Janice Smith's foot, were a major problem at the hospital for which I worked. Diabetic patients, many whose blood sugar was poorly controlled, regularly presented to our emergency room with deep foot infections. It seemed that once or twice a week, this type of patient was admitted

---

[130] Losing hospital beds can have significant financial implications for the individual surgeons—and create marked inconvenience for the patients they have scheduled for surgery. If a service (orthopaedics, vascular, etc.) has filled all of its allotted hospital beds, surgeons on that service are not allowed to perform elective operations that require admission to hospital after surgery. These elective surgical cases then need to be canceled, and these patients, who have often been waiting months, need to be rescheduled. This is a great inconvenience to the affected patient, and a source of tremendous frustration for the surgeon. Furthermore, the operating room time usually cannot be rescheduled on such short notice to accommodate a surgical patient who does not need to be admitted. Therefore, the surgeon loses the money he or she would normally have received for performing the cancelled elective surgery. This money is substantial and cannot be recouped. This is one of the primary reasons surgeons argue: over which service emergency patients get admitted to. These decisions indirectly take money out of the pockets of individual surgeons.

through our emergency room. Sometimes the foot could be salvaged; sometimes it could not. Often, an argument with the vascular service would ensue—the same argument over hospital beds that I witnessed twenty years ago as an intern.

Perhaps our hospital, by the nature of its patient population, saw a disproportionate number of diabetic foot infections. However, I have no doubt this was also a problem at almost all other hospitals. The effect of diabetes was a ubiquitous problem.

Canada, the country where Sir Fredrick Banting discovered the first effective treatment for diabetics, was ideally positioned to treat these patients in a proactive, cost-effective manner. If Janice Smith, and other diabetic patients like her, could have been seen regularly and screened for foot ulcerations, it is much less likely that she would have ended up in the emergency room. She would not have spent two weeks in the hospital, undergoing multiple surgeries. She would not have required the services of high-priced surgeons. And she likely would not have lost her leg.

Like many conditions in medicine, an ounce of prevention is worth a pound of cure. Medical literature is replete with studies, demonstrating the beneficial effects of preventive treatment for patients with diabetes.[131,132] There are clear, evidence-based algorithms outlining how patients should be educated and screened to minimize the risk of developing the end results of diabetes: loss of sight, renal failure, and serious foot infections leading to amputation.[133]

Canada's single-payer healthcare system—where every patient has insurance, and there is central oversight of the system—was ideally set up to develop a proactive, region-wide diabetic foot screening and treatment program. A year after returning to Canada, I attempted to develop and institute such a program. My goal was to proactively

---

[131] Singh N, Armstrong DG, Lipsky BA. "Preventing foot ulcers in patients with diabetes." JAMA. 2005 Jan 12. 293(2):217-28.

[132] "Guideline for management of wounds in patients with lower-extremity neuropathic disease." *WOCN Guidelines*. (http://www.guideline.gov/content. aspx?id=38248)

[133] Preventive Foot Care in Diabetes. American Diabetes Association.http:// care.diabetesjournals.org/content/27/suppl_1/s63.full

minimize the number of serious foot infections in our hospital emergency room. Ending the long-standing turf battle between the orthopaedic and vascular surgery services would be an additional bonus.

I contacted the head of the provincial health ministry's newly-introduced Activity-Based Funding (ABF) program and arranged a meeting. I explained the problem and outlined a straightforward, algorithmically-based preventive program. It was designed not just to help the diabetic patients at my hospital, but throughout the entire health region. He was enamored and said this was exactly the type of program they were looking to support. He said that funding of between $800,000 and $1.2 million would seem reasonable, provided we could document the benefits over the existing situation. I wrote a proposal for $650,000 and submitted it to the administrative head of our hospital's surgery program. She reviewed it and then simply said this was not something the hospital was interested in doing.

Perhaps from the hospital's point of view, this program did not make sense. Maybe they were concerned that any attempt to provide coordinated management of diabetic patients would indirectly attract this patient population to our hospital—a population that has traditionally used a disproportionate amount of hospital resources. Each hospital has its own agenda—an agenda that is often at odds with the goals of the health region and the provincial ministry of health. Most importantly, hospital agendas are almost never formally aligned with the healthcare needs of the population. Whatever the reason, for Janice Smith and all the other diabetic patients (as well as the taxpayers of the province), a coordinated diabetic foot management program was desperately needed, and yet it could not find a home anywhere in the healthcare system.

The type of proactive diabetic screening and treatment program just described is an example of a program that fulfills the *Triple Aim*. The *triple aim* is a concept promoted by Donald Berwick, President of the Institute for Healthcare Improvement (IHI) and one of the primary architects of the IOM's *Crossing the Quality Chasm*. The *triple aim* highlights the simultaneous goals of 1) improving the quality of care including the patient's experience, 2) improving the health of specific populations, and 3) decreasing the per capita cost of healthcare.[134] To the uninitiated, these goals might seem to be in conflict. How can care be improved, while at the same time substantially decreasing the cost? The answer is that the waste in a healthcare system like Canada's leaves substantial opportunities to implement *triple aim* projects.

Consider Janice Smith. The quality of care, and her resulting experience, would have been dramatically improved had she been able to receive regular, low-cost screening and basic treatment for her diabetic foot condition—before it became affected by an unsalvageable infection. Focusing on the larger population of diabetics as a whole allows for the implementation of coordinated, systematic, and relatively low-cost interventions at a much earlier stage.

This was one of the unique features of the *triple aim*—a renewed emphasis on defined populations. Dramatic, per capita cost-saving can be achieved when validated, evidence-based screening and treatment protocols are applied to specific populations, fulfilling the third arm of the *triple aim*. The Canadian healthcare system, with its universal insurance and central oversight, should in theory be positioned to implement programs that fulfill the *triple aim*. However, the historical structure of the system, as outlined in Chapter 5, makes widespread implementation of these types of programs practically impossible in most healthcare settings.

Tools for Standardizing and Improving Medical Care: The Checklist

Do you know what medical advance has saved the most lives (and money) in the 21st century? In one of the most important medicine-related articles written this century (and in a non-medical publication no less), Dr. Atul Gawande described the stunning benefits of systematizing medical care. His article, "The Checklist," was published in *The New*

---

[134] Berwick DM, Nolan TW, Whittington J. "The Triple Aim: Care, Health, and Cost." *Health Affairs*. May 2008. Vol 27(3): 759-769

Yorker on December 7, 2007.[135] It outlines Dr. Peter Pronovost's simple solution for decreasing (i.e., practically eliminating) life-threatening, central line infections in patients admitted to intensive care units (ICUs).

Pronovost, an ICU attending physician at Johns Hopkins Medical Center in Baltimore, had become alarmed by the devastating effect that infections stemming from contaminated intravenous lines had on the seriously ill and injured patients who had been admitted to his ICU. In ICU patients, these so-called *line infections* increased the mortality rate significantly—and the length of stay by an average of seven days for those patients who did survive.

Central line infections, at the time Pronovost began studying them, were not actually that common, occurring at a rate of only 1.8-5.2 per 1000 catheter days.[136,137]However, uncommon things happen commonly when there are enough events, and this was certainly the case with busy ICUs. A typical 15- to 30-bed ICU at a large hospital, such as the one I worked at in Canada, would have 500-1000 ICU admissions per year. Something that happened "only" 3% of the time could easily affect 30 patients a year.

How could these infections be eliminated? That was the question Pronovost faced. Line infections tended to occur when the intravenous line was placed in a non-sterile manner, or when the line was kept in for too many days. This information had been known for decades, along with the solution to this problem. Pronovost established a systematic

---

[135] The Checklist: If something so simple can transform intensive care, what else can it do? By Atul Gawande. *The New Yorker.* December 10th 20007. http://www.newyorker.com/magazine/2007/12/10/the-checklist (Accessed December 24th, 2015.)

[136] O'Grady NP, Alexander M, Dellinger EP, et al. "Guidelines for the prevention of intravascular catheter-related infections." *MMWR Recomm Rep.* 2002. 51(RR-10): 1-29.

[137] "National Nosocomial Infections Surveillance System." *National Nosocomial Infection Surveillance (NNIS) system report.* Data summary from 1992 through June 2004, issued October 2004. Am J of Inf Control. 32: 470-85.

process, beginning in 1998, to ensure that *every* patient in the ICU at Johns Hopkins would get appropriate line management.[138]

He developed a five-step checklist for doctors to follow when inserting a central intravenous line:

(1) Doctors were to thoroughly wash their hands with antibacterial soap.
(2) The patient's skin was to be cleaned with chlorhexidine antiseptic.
(3) Sterile drapes were to be placed over the entire patient.
(4) Doctors were to wear a sterile mask, hat, gown, and gloves.
(5) A sterile dressing was to be applied over the catheter once it had been inserted. To this list, he added a plan to ensure the central line was either removed or changed within five days.

Every ICU doctor more or less knew this was what should be done; the hard part was getting physicians to actually do this when they inserted a central line. To achieve this goal, Pronovost enlisted the ICU nursing staff to actually go through the checklist with the physician when the central line was being inserted. Initially, there was notable resistance, as the physicians considered themselves *experts*, and some felt that this approach was demeaning to their skills and judgment. Once instituted, the results were unequivocal. In the first year of use, the ICU at Johns Hopkins did not have a single central line infection. However, would it work at other—perhaps more chaotic—centres?

In 2003, the Michigan Health and Hospital Association asked Pronovost if he could introduce his checklist program for use within its

---

[138] Berenholtz SM, Pronovost PJ, Lipsett PA, Hobson D, Earsing K, Farley JE, Milanovich S, Garrett-Mayer E, Winters BD, Rubin HR, Dorman T, Perl TM. "Eliminating catheter-related bloodstream infections in the intensive care unit."*Crit Care Med.* 2004 Oct. 32(10):2014-20.

ICUs, which included over 100 Michigan hospitals.[139] Many of these hospitals were in low-income districts, such as the Detroit metropolitan area. Many were losing money, and morale among the staff was low.

Pronovost helped introduce a program aimed at systematizing the care that was provided in these ICUs. They called it the Keystone Initiative. It involved standardizing certain procedures via checklists. It also involved enlisting the help of hospital executives by demanding that each hospital unit that was part of the study have a hospital executive assigned to that ward, in order to help facilitate any needed changes.

Published in the *New England Journal of Medicine* in 2006, the results of the Keystone Initiative were staggering.[140] The simple checklists, and the other basic strategies they had employed to systematize care delivery in the Michigan ICUs, had decreased the catheter-related infection rate by 66%. By one estimate, they saved 1500 lives and $175 million in the first 18 months of the program.[141]

Gawande's article on The Checklist introduced to the public what he, Pronovost, and others had been doing to improve standardization of medical care and decrease the variation in the delivery of treatment. The checklist technique he presents is just one of many tools available to systematize care delivery. Standardizing the approach to care in no way implies that the judgment of physicians, nurses, and other healthcare professionals will no longer be necessary. However, standardizing baseline care processes can save millions of dollars and, more importantly, thousands of patients' lives.

---

[139] "In addition to the intervention to reduce the rate of catheter-related bloodstream infection, the ICUs implemented the use of daily goal sheets to improve clinician-to-clinician communication within the ICU, an intervention to reduce the incidence of ventilator-related pneumonia, and a comprehensive unit-based safety program to improve the safety culture." Excerpted from *NEJM* 355(26): December 28, 2006.

[140] Pronovost P, Needham D, Bernholtz S, et al. "An intervention to reduce catheter-related bloodstream infections in the ICU." *N Engl J Med.* 2006. 355:2725-32.

[141] The Checklist: If something so simple can transform intensive care, what else can it do? By Atul Gawande. *The New Yorker.* December 10th 20007. http://www.newyorker.com/magazine/2007/12/10/the-checklist (Accessed December 24th, 2015.)

Quality and Process Improvement Initiatives

"Really, does it take all that to figure out what house movers, wedding planners, and tax accountants figured out ages ago?" Gawande asked, referring to Provonost's huge research study demonstrating the profound benefits of the ICU checklist initiative. Sadly, the answer is *yes*—and probably more. Physicians and administrators have learned *how things are done* via role modeling from more experienced colleagues throughout their years of training. They do not easily embrace new and fundamentally different ways of delivering care. Until recently, the process by which care is delivered has largely been ignored.

Pronovost summed it up best when he described the *three buckets of healthcare*. The *first bucket* is understanding biology: being able to identify what diseases and injuries are affecting the patient. On the whole, medicine does this very well. The *second bucket* is developing effective treatment. This is also done fairly well, although not always with curative results. The *third bucket* is "ensuring that those therapies are delivered effectively."[142]

This *third bucket* is what checklist initiatives, and other quality and process improvement tools designed to systematize care, aim to address. This is where the work needs to be done. It is where the really dramatic improvements in healthcare will come in the next few decades. An intense focus on standardizing and improving the actual care delivery process will be the defining feature of the *era of systematized medicine*. Yet this approach of focusing on reforming the care delivery process is still largely being ignored within much of the Canadian healthcare system.

"I am so frustrated that no one in the operating room performs the pre-surgical checklist correctly!" This was a comment I made to Jennifer Jefferson, the administrative head of the surgical program, during one of our monthly one-on-one meetings—in my role as the head of the orthopaedic department.

"What do you mean?" she asked.

---

[142] Gawande, Atul (December 2007). "The Checklist, If something so simple can transform intensive care, what else can it do?". New Yorker Magazine. p. 86. (Accessed December 24th 2015).

"The pre-surgical checklist before we start an operation…. No one does it correctly!"

"I don't understand," Jennifer reiterated. I started to restate my frustration for a third time, but she had already turned to her computer and, with a few clicks of her mouse, had brought up a document. "Look, Steve, here is the operating room checklist data for the last two years. We have a 100% compliance rate with the pre-surgical checklist during that time period."

"Really?" I asked. "So that data includes the two patients where members of our department operated on the wrong extremity?"

Like many healthcare administrators, Jennifer was divorced from the healthcare playing field and had made the mistake that so many administrators make time and time again. She placed too much weight on data that shows up on her computer screen—data that usually does not fully represent what is actually happening. I was correct, but so was she. Our hospital was not doing the checklist prior to surgery correctly. We were missing many steps, and most individuals involved did not begin to understand the purpose of the pre-surgical checklist. However, Jennifer was also correct; we had done a checklist (of some sort) prior to every surgery.

This illustrates the difficulty in instituting process improvement. It is not just enough to introduce a process improvement tool like a pre-surgical checklist; it needs to be done correctly—every time. This takes buy-in and engagement from everyone involved, and that can be a huge challenge.

Decreasing variation in a complex production process improves quality.[143,144] This is an accepted core principle of business. The same concept can be applied directly to medical care. Decreasing the variation

---

[143] "What is the Law of Variation?" American Society for Quality website. Based on Timothy J. Clark's *Success Through Quality: Support Guide for the Journey to Continuous Improvement*, ASQ Quality Press, 1999. http://asq.org/learn-about-quality/variation/overview/overview.html (Accessed April 28, 2015.)

[144] 14 Key Principles from *Out of the Crisis* by W. Edwards Deming. Cambridge, MA: Massachusetts Institute of Technology, Center for Advanced Engineering Study, ©1986. http://en.wikipedia.org/wiki/W. Edwards Deming (Accessed April 28, 2015.)

that occurs in an event that is repeated over and over again (such as a surgical episode of care) is one of the hallmarks of the quality improvement movement. As Pronovost and others have demonstrated, well-developed and appropriately-implemented checklists are one method of decreasing variation.

Checklists are merely tools—one of many tools that have been developed to help systematize and standardize medical care delivery. When used appropriately, these tools can dramatically improve the quality of medical care that is delivered.

Lean thinking and the *Six Sigma* process are examples of quality improvement tools that were developed in other industries and have recently been applied to the medical system with success. *Lean thinking* was developed by Toyota and *Six Sigma* was pioneered at Motorola before being popularized by General Electric.[145,146] A variety of other quality and process improvement tools have been developed and may be applied to the practice of medicine (See Table 3), including care paths, clinical practice guidelines, total quality management, patient and family centred care (PFCC), root cause analysis, and failure modes and effects analysis (FMEA). All of the tools summarized in Table 3 have been designed to either standardize or improve the process of care delivery. When implemented successfully, they have been shown to significantly improve the quality—and decrease the cost—of care that is delivered.

---

[145] Womack, James P., Daniel, T. Jones (1996) Lean Thinking

[146] Adams, Cary W.; Gupta, Praveen; Wilson, Charles E. (2003). Six Sigma Deployment. Burlington, MA: Butterworth-Heinemann.

Table 3: Summary of Quality and Process Improvement Tools[147]

Quality & Process Improvement Tools	Description
Checklist Initiatives	Standardizes and improves team communication around a specific event by formally reviewing a preset checklist
Clinical Practice Guidelines (CPGs)	Formal guidelines for diagnosis or management of a clinical situation that are usually generated in an evidence-based manner
Appropriate Use Criteria (AUCs)	Guidelines developed based on the collective judgment of experts on the appropriateness of various diagnostic testing and treatment options in specific clinical scenarios
Care Pathways (Clinical Pathways, Care Map)	A formal pathway that outlines how care for a specific condition is to be delivered throughout the entire EOC
Standardized Clinical Assessment and Management Plan (SCAMP)	A care path developed with increased emphasis on the use of evidence-based literature and employing real-time feedback and data analysis, allowing for regular changes to the pathway as needed
Plan-Do-Check-Act (PDCA) Cycles	A four-step, iterative, continuous improvement cycle that envisions what the process should look like ("Plan"); implements the Plan ("Do"); records the results ("Check"); and adjusts the process based on the results ("Act")
Statistical Quality Control (SQC)	The use of outcome or output data collected as part of the production process to continuously improve the process and provide early detection of problems
Lean Process Improvement	A multidisciplinary, team-based process for improving value and flow in the provision of services that was developed by the Toyota Motor company

---

[147] Excerpted with permission from Table 3. Pinney SJ, Page AE, Jevsevar DS, Bozic K. Current Concept review: Quality and Process Improvement in Orthopedics. *Orthopedic Research and Reviews.* Dovepress Volume 2016: 8 pages 1-11. December 23rd 2015 http://dx.doi.org/10.2147/ORR.S92216.

Six Sigma	A process improvement strategy introduced by the Motorola company that focuses on 1) decreasing the rate that defects (errors) occur, and 2) reducing variation in the production process
Lean Six Sigma	An amalgamation of the principles of *lean thinking* (eliminating waste and improving workflow) and *six sigma* (decreasing the rate of errors and reducing process variation)
Total Quality Management (TQM)	A comprehensive approach to continuous quality improvement of the entire process involving all members of the health care team including patients.
Patient and Family Centered Care Methodology (PFCC)	A six-step, continuous improvement process developed specifically for healthcare based on TQM principles
Root Cause Analysis (RCA)	A formalized approach to evaluating the cause or causes of an adverse event.
Failure Modes and Effects Analysis (FMEA)	A proactive approach to preventing adverse events by identifying potential failure modes within the existing system.

EOC = episode of care

The *triple aim* has clarified the mission of the modern medical system in simplified terms. Quality and process improvement tools such as checklist initiatives provide the means by which the system can evolve to meet the goals of the *triple aim*. In many instances, including within the Canadian healthcare system, the underlying foundation on which the system is built makes the full incorporation of these initiatives difficult or impossible.

Michael Porter: Applying Business Strategies to Healthcare

The growing recognition that healthcare delivery needed to be fundamentally redesigned may have been crystallized by the IOM's publication of *Crossing the Quality Chasm* and the identification of the *triple aim*. However, the details of what this new system might look like and how the transition may occur in specific jurisdictions were still not clear. One of the most respected and viable proposals for health system reform originated from Harvard Business School Professor Michael Porter and his colleagues. Incorporating many of the principles proposed in the IOM's report, Porter outlined his view of what a modern medical system should look like in his book *Redefining Health Care*, as well as a series of papers—including "The Strategy That Will Fix Health Care," which was published in the *Harvard Business Review*.[148,149,150]

Porter's central thesis is that a modern healthcare system should focus on "maximizing value for patients." He defines value as the "best outcomes at the lowest cost."[151] Porter repeatedly emphasizes the need to focus on quality healthcare. Merely lowering the cost without ensuring high quality does not optimize the value equation. A move towards a *value-based* healthcare system demands a move away from the existing *volume-oriented* system, where practitioners and institutions are paid based on the specific procedures and interventions that are performed. In a value-based system, the ultimate results of the care are compensated, not the individual elements.

Value-based care means paying for healthcare outputs, not inputs.[152] In this case, *outputs* are the final results of care: a successful surgical episode of care, a certain number of primary care patients managed effectively over a set period of time, or a chronic disease, such as renal failure, successfully treated over a defined period. Traditional healthcare *inputs* are doctors' visits, isolated surgical procedures, and investigations, such as blood tests and MRIs. These types of inputs are often essential for delivering effective care, but Porter argues that they should not be reimbursed in isolation from the end results. Yet this is exactly what the present, fee-for-service system does.

---

148 Porter ME and Olmstead-Teisberg E. *Redefining Health Care: Creating Value-Based Competition on Results*. Harvard Business School Publishing. 2006.

149 Porter ME and Lee TH. "The Strategy That Will Fix Health Care." *Harvard Business Review*. October 2013: p. 50-70.

150 Porter ME. "What is value in healthcare?" *N Engl J Med*. 2010. 363(26): 2477-81

151 Porter ME and Lee TH. "The Strategy That Will Fix Health Care." *Harvard Business Review*. October 2013: p. 51.

152 Porter ME. "What is value in healthcare?" *N Engl J Med*. 2010. 363(26): 2477-81.

Porter's focus on value in the care that is *actually* delivered represents a radical departure from how most healthcare systems are organized—including the Canadian system. Operationalizing his ideas requires a fundamentally different way of organizing care—and a plan for how the transition from one system to another can be brought about. Porter has outlined a six-step *value agenda* that would characterize this new, value-based healthcare system. With respect to the difficult transition from an existing system to a new system, he recommended that financial incentives be reorganized to facilitate required changes. In Canada, this would entail fundamental system reorganization; one model of the type of reorganization envisioned will be outlined in Chapter 9.

"Define the goal!" Even before outlining his six-step *value agenda*, Porter emphasized the need to define the end goal of any healthcare system. Understanding the end goal of any system seems like a self-evident statement; however, for many healthcare systems, there is often no clear, specific set of goals that have been defined. General goals, such as "providing high-quality, patient-centred care," are often listed, but they serve only as aspirational statements. Delineating population-based healthcare needs is essential —along with identifying corresponding outcomes that are specific, clear, and can be accurately measured. Without an orientation to specific end goals, a system will meander aimlessly, wasting resources and falling far short of its potential effectiveness.

The six components of Porter's value agenda are as follows:

1. Organize into integrated practice units (IPUs).
2. Measure outcomes and costs for every patient.
3. Move to bundled payments for care cycles.
4. Integrate care delivery across separate facilities.
5. Expand excellent services across geography.
6. Build an enabling information technology platform.

These were not designed as isolated components. Rather, Porter emphasized the need for them to be completely interdependent and mutually reinforcing. A basic understanding of these six components and how they would transform a healthcare system is essential.

1. Organize into Integrated Practice Units (IPUs)

Creating IPUs essentially means creating teams. This requires undoing the existing, siloed organization of medicine and reorienting care around the needs of the patient. It represents true, *patient-centred care*. Rather than maintaining specialized departments, such as surgery, medicine, anesthesia, and nursing, Porter proposes that care delivery be organized around patients and their conditions, such as IPUs for cancer, musculoskeletal conditions, renal failure, and eye disorders. At the heart of the healthcare system would be IPU teams organized to provide comprehensive primary care to patients. IPU teams would not only diagnose and provide care, they would also "assume responsibility for engaging patients and their families in care—for instance, by providing education and counseling."[153] All IPU personnel would work together toward common goals, and communication would flow freely between all members of the team.

2. Measure Outcomes and Costs for Every Patient

Accurate outcome measures are one of the cornerstones of modern medicine. In order to improve the results of care, the actual results that are presently being provided needs to be fully understood. This statement seems obvious. In fact, one of North America's early orthopaedic surgeons Dr. Ernest Codman proposed the "end results idea" in 1910:[154]

> "*The common sense notion that every hospital should follow every patient it treats, long enough to determine whether or not the treatment has been successful, and then to inquire, 'If not, why not?' With a view to preventing similar failures in the future.*"

---

[153] Porter ME, Lee TH. *The Strategy That Will Fix Health Care*. Harvard Business Review. October 2013: p. 53.

[154] Donabedian A: The end results of health care: Ernest Codman's contribution to quality assessment and beyond. *Milbank Quarterly*, 67(2): 233-256, 1989.

As intuitive as this idea might be, it has not been incorporated with any sort of regularity or accuracy in traditional medical practices. Porter, like others, including those from the IOM, emphasizes the critical need to have accurate outcome data. This includes generating accurate answers to the following types of questions:

- How do patients fare following the treatment they received (*clinical outcomes*)?
- What is the complication rate of the various treatments that are administered (*complication rate*)?
- How satisfied are the patients with the treatment they received (*patient satisfaction*)?
- What were the costs of the treatment (*per capita cost*)?

This outcome data needs to be reviewed over the entire cycle of care. Furthermore, collection of this data needs to be independent and unbiased—and built into the entire process. Accurate outcome data allows appropriate feedback loops to be created to improve the existing healthcare system. Finally, accurate outcome metrics are an essential element of ensuring accountability in those who are responsible for leading the healthcare system.

3. Move to Bundled Payments for Care Cycles

The method by which healthcare is funded drives how healthcare is delivered. Porter argues that *bundled payments* are the only effective means for tying payments to both quality and cost-effectiveness. Bundled payments are payments that cover the entire episode of care (or care cycle) for acute conditions (and for management of chronic conditions for a defined period of time). Bundled payments are payments not merely for the delivery of care, but for the delivery of care that meets certain standards, including outcomes, complication rates, and patient satisfaction scores.

Unlike fee-for-service payments (which reward high-volume care) and global capitation payments (which reward rationing care), *bundled payments* reward value. They force a realignment of healthcare delivery along a team-based approach to ensure that all providers are working toward a common goal. Bundled payments also force the delivery system to be constantly evaluated; when this occurs, dramatic savings can often be realized as unnecessary and expensive resources are identified and eliminated.

4. Integrate Care Delivery Systems

Porter argues for moving away from standalone hospitals that provide a full range of services in each community. Instead, he recommends eliminating fragmentation and duplication of care by integrating care for patients across locations. For example, there would no longer be competing orthopaedic; ear, nose, and throat (ENT); and thoracic surgery departments at three separate, neighboring hospitals. Rather, integrating care would demand that all orthopedic service lines be centred at one hospital, ENT care at another, and thoracic care at a third. Quality and cost-effectiveness tend to improve noticeably as volume in a particular area increases.

5. Expand Geographic Reach

To increase value further, Porter argues that large, integrated healthcare systems—with an expanded reach—need to be developed. One way of doing this is to have a hub-and-spoke setup, whereby a major, centralized medical centre provides high-level, complex care— with routine, less expensive care being provided at a series of satellite offices or hospitals. The central oversight of the healthcare system in Canada, both at the Ministry of Health level and via Health Regions, offers the opportunity to institute a more coordinated, geographical approach to healthcare delivery. In some instances, this is being done relatively successfully. For example, cardiac care in the province of British Columbia occurs at one of four centres. However, as was illustrated in Chapter 5, the historical structure of the Canadian healthcare system means that most hospitals tend to remain *full service*—a philosophical approach that dilutes expertise and undermines value.

6. *Build an Enabling Information Technology Platform*

Communication is critical in healthcare delivery, yet it has been woefully inadequate in traditional healthcare systems. Paper charts full of illegible writing— and an almost complete inability to exchange healthcare information between hospitals—has been the norm. Information technology that is centred around patient needs offers the opportunity to dramatically improve communication—and by extension, quality of care—within a coordinated healthcare system. Porter proposes an IT platform that is centred on patients, uses common data definitions, encompasses all types of patient data, is accessible to all parties involved in care, includes templates for standard care paths for each medical condition, and makes the extraction of outcome information easy.

Such an IT system, interwoven throughout the delivery system, would serve to dramatically transform care. This has already happened in many systems, including the Mayo Clinic, the Cleveland Clinic, and Kaiser Permanente in California. In theory, it could happen in Canada, given that the mandates for care originate with each provincial government. However, while there have been programs to promote increased use of electronic medical records, there has not been a mandate to ensure this occurs in a coordinated, systematic manner.

Summary: Chapter 6

The IOM called for a fundamental reform of the way healthcare is delivered. Donald Berwick outlined the *triple aim* of improving the quality of care, improving the health of specific populations, and decreasing the cost of healthcare. Atul Gawande, Peter Pronovost, and others have demonstrated the profound benefit of systematizing care by the use of process improvement tools, such as checklist initiatives designed to decrease variations in care and minimize errors. Michael Porter and his colleagues outlined a clear framework of what it looks like for a modern healthcare system to optimize value—the best patient outcomes at the lowest cost.

These are not specifically Canadian ideas. Good healthcare does not have national borders. The principles derived from these and other ideas are just as relevant within the Canadian healthcare system as they are in any other, first-world health system. However, to invoke these ideas means a fundamental paradigm shift in how healthcare is delivered. Is Canada ready for this type of change?

Steven Lewis, one of Canada's foremost healthcare consultants, summarized the need for these types of changes in a 2007 commentary[155]:

> *"What's truly unsustainable is doing business the same old way. We cannot continue to consume expensive new drugs when less expensive older ones are just as effective most of the time. We cannot continue to have specialists do what family doctors ought to do, family doctors do what nurse practitioners ought to do and nurses do what licensed practical nurses ought to do. We cannot persist with a voluntarist, incremental model of quality improvement, where practitioners and institutions are free to embrace or refuse to adopt smarter and cheaper ways of delivering care. We cannot continue to accept the price of goods and services that have no relationship to what they deliver."*

Let's return to the hockey scenario at the start of this chapter. Why did the NHL all-stars lose to the Soviet Union? Why doesn't having the best players ensure you will have the best team?

The principles of organizing a high-quality, modern medical system, such as those outlined in this chapter, are similar to the principles of running an outstanding hockey team. In both situations, there are common elements, and there is the need to embrace certain philosophies and adhere to certain principles. Many of these ideas are self-evident and have long been ingrained in running a professional hockey team. Yet these elements were often absent or incomplete in the Canadian healthcare system I witnessed.

---

[155] Steven Lewis. Commentary in *Healthcare Quarterly.* 2007.Vol 10 (2): 103.

Four core ideas—pillars of the system—are critical, whether the goal is leading a Stanley Cup-winning hockey team or running an effective healthcare system that truly serves the patients and the taxpayers.

1. Have clear goals.

What are the goals of your team? What are the goals of your healthcare system? Make sure goals are very specific, not just aspirational (e.g., to win games or to provide high-quality care). Without a clear destination, how can a hockey team or a healthcare system expect to get to where it needs to be?

2. Work as a team to achieve patient-centred goals.

In hockey, this means ensuring that all players are working in unison, and at their highest level, toward the goal of winning each game. In healthcare, it means being truly *patient-centred*—working as a team to provide high-quality and high-value care to the patients that flow through the system. Just as a hockey team needs to focus on what elements lead to victory, healthcare systems need to focus on what needs to happen to each patient in order for them to have success. This demands viewing healthcare delivery from the patient's perspective.

3. Accurately measure the results (and act on the results).

In professional hockey, results matter; the standings are published each day in the newspaper. It is clear for everyone to see which teams are winning games, and ultimately which team wins the Stanley Cup. Results are even more important in healthcare. Accurately measuring the outcomes of care, and acting on the subsequent results, is one of the pillars of the new healthcare delivery paradigm. Yet unlike hockey, medicine has traditionally done a poor job of accurately measuring the results of care. Detailed measures are required.

In today's professional hockey, much more than wins and losses are recorded. Power play efficiency, penalty-killing effectiveness, and the ability to hold a lead in the third period are just a few of the many metrics that are recorded for an NHL hockey team. Similarly, the performances of individual players are measured. Playing time, plus/ minus status, and more advanced metrics (such as location-specific shooting percentage) are used to analyze the effectiveness of teams and players.[156] Accurate metrics allow coaches and general managers—those running the teams—to make informed decisions to improve their team's overall performance.

As Porter outlines in the second component of his *value agenda*, healthcare systems need to collect a variety of accurate and detailed metrics to assess the overall results of care, patient satisfaction, complication rates, and the cost of care. Without these accurate metrics collected as a part of the care delivery process, those running the healthcare system will not be able to identify problematic areas, and subsequently implement quality and process improvement programs to optimize care. The ICU catheter initiative undertaken by Peter Pronovost is just one example of the benefits of accurately measuring the results of care.

4. Pay for outputs, not inputs.

Hockey teams organize their rosters in a way that the managers believe will optimize their chance for on-ice success. Hockey teams cannot buy guaranteed success, but *buying* success is exactly what they are attempting to do when they sign players to contracts. Before offering a player a contract, the general manager needs to make a complicated assessment as to the overall value of that player's contributions to the team winning. A player may be an *input*, but the general manager is indirectly trying to pay for an *output*—winning. The general manager's job depends on getting these assessments correct.

Similarly, the healthcare system needs to focus on paying for the results of care—outputs. This is the concept behind the movement toward bundled payments and care cycles. It is akin to paying for the results of a hockey game, not merely the constituent parts, which is what presently occurs. Implicit in this movement is the need to fundamentally reform the manner in which the Canadian healthcare

---

[156] http://hockeymetrics.net

system funds care—and the recognition that those managers who get this equation wrong need to be held accountable, in the same manner that hockey managers are ultimately held accountable when their team underperforms.

These four core pillars, when consistently applied to a healthcare system, form a foundation for providing high-value, modern medical care. There are numerous other principles that also need to be invoked in order to consistently achieve success in complex endeavours such as hockey and healthcare including:

- Continuously improve team performance based on feedback.
- Decrease variation in a process to improve the end results.
- Hold individuals accountable for their work performance.
- Have clear team/organization leadership that is intimately connected with the workplace *playing field*.
- Reward excellence and penalize detrimental behaviours.
- These are but a few of the known principles for success. Many of these principles are self-evident. Others have been validated in other industries.

Hockey teams know that a failure to meet one or more of these principles will undermine their ability to be successful, and, in many instances, it is a prescription for failure. Within the Canadian healthcare system, the relative lack of system accountability has meant that many of these principles have been ignored for decades. The next chapter will review the existing structure of the Canadian healthcare system and will contrast this with how a modern healthcare system is structured in general terms. Chapter 8 will then review in more detail the specific principles that each area within the healthcare system must embrace.

<u>Summary Points: Chapter 6</u>

By the year 2000 continued marked variations in care and the persistence of large numbers of medical errors lead healthcare experts to conclude that the traditional healthcare system needed to be fundamentally reformed.

Most medical errors were deemed to be *system errors* the product of the fragmented, siloed nature of how care delivery was organized.

The concept of the *triple aim* was proposed to highlight three simultaneous goals of modern healthcare: 1) improve the quality of care provided, 2) improve the health of specific populations, and 3) decrease the per capita cost of health care.

Improving the standardization of medical care has demonstrated a decrease in treatment variation with improved overall results –often at a lower cost. The use of checklist initiatives is just one of many quality and process improvement tools available to help systematize healthcare delivery.

Modern healthcare systems should focus on maximizing value for patients with value defined as the "best outcome at the lowest cost."

Four core pillars of a high functioning modern healthcare system were proposed:

1. Have clear goals
2. Work as a team to achieve patient centred goals
3. Accurately measure the results of care –and act on these results
4. Pay for outputs, not inputs

CHAPTER 7

Contrasting Models for Healthcare Delivery in Canada

In March 1914, the Toronto Hockey Club, league champions of the National Hockey Association (NHA), defeated the Pacific Coast Hockey Association (PCHA) league champions, the Victoria Aristocrats, 3 games to 0 to defend the Stanley Cup. One hundred years later, the Los Angeles Kings survived an arduous journey through four best-of-seven playoff rounds—after an 82-game regular season—to capture the Stanley Cup. Winning the Stanley Cup was one of the few things these teams had in common, as the nature and organization of the game of hockey had changed radically over the intervening century.

A direct comparison of the games from the 1914 and 2014 Stanley Cup championships would be striking. In 1914, forward passes were illegal, and the equipment was rudimentary. Each team only had nine players, and substitutions were rare, meaning most players played the entire game. In contrast, by 2014, forward passes were legal, and sticks were curved and made of strong, high-tech material. Each team dressed 18 players (plus two goalies); the average shift lasted about 45 seconds.[158] In 2014, games were fast, exciting, and predicated on intricate teamwork in order to achieve success.

---

[157]   http://www.arcticicehockey.com/2010/2/10/1270271/
         shift-length-change-since-1997-98

In the 1914 Stanley Cup Challenge, two competing leagues had distinctly different rules. NHA rules were used in the first and third games. The second of the three games was played using PCHA rules, which allowed seven players on the ice—including the now-extinct position of rover. In 2014, the National Hockey League (NHL) was still evaluating the rules of hockey regularly, but the core rules of passing, penalties, and offside had been stable for many years. The NHL regularly reviewed the league schedule, the rules of the game, and the playoff format to ensure that the game of hockey was exciting and fair—and that the league as a whole prospered.

Introduction: Structure Dictates Function

The central thesis of this book is that the Canadian healthcare system needs fundamental reform to ensure long-term sustainability. The means to this reform is a structural reorganization to align the care delivery process with accepted, basic principles of running a modern, systematized medical system. These ideas, including the four foundational pillars (Table 4), were outlined in the previous chapter and will be expanded upon in Chapter 8. They have been delineated by organizations like the *Institute of Medicine*, as well as healthcare thought leaders like Donald Berwick, Atul Gawande, Peter Pronovost, Michael Porter, and Stephen Lewis. As important as these guiding principles might be in reality, most of these ideas are largely just common sense.

Yet, because of the history of how medicine has evolved in Canada, as outlined in Chapter 5, the resulting rigidity of the existing organizational structure precludes many of these ideas from being easily instituted. This is not to imply that there are no pockets of excellence within the present system. There are examples where individuals and groups have worked *around* the existing infrastructure to render excellent care based on these principles. However, to do this often requires extraordinary effort and a series of *workarounds*, rather than a direct route to implementing these ideas. The structure of an organization usually dictates how it will function—and the Canadian medical system is no exception.

Table 4: Four Foundational Pillars for a Modern Healthcare System

> 1. **Have clear goals.** Know what each part of the system needs to be doing, and how it relates to the larger system.
> 2. **Work as a team to achieve patient-centred goals.** Understanding the needs of patients as they flow through a health system allows appropriate teams to be formed to address these needs. Forming teams that work together in a coordinated manner—to optimally serve the patients they are treating—is critical to improving the quality and efficiency of patient care.

3. **Accurately measure the results of care—and act on the results.** All core aspects of patient care need to be accurately measured within a health system. Based on these ongoing results, feedback loops must be built into the system to continually improve care on an iterative basis.

4. **Pay for outputs, not inputs.** How a healthcare system is funded determines how it is organized. Funding should pay for the outputs of the system: successful episodes of care or patients appropriately managed over a set period of time. Doctors, nurses, administrators, and medical equipment are all examples of inputs to the medical system. They are all essential for the effective running of the system, but they should not be paid for in insolation of results.

Journeying Through the Canadian Healthcare System

What follows is a story that contrasts the existing means by which healthcare is typically delivered in Canada with a model for care delivery based on foundational principles. Through this analysis, a better understanding of what modern healthcare delivery actually looks like will emerge.

Christopher Barclay's medical adventure began one Saturday in April. He was a healthy 47-year-old who, while painting the spare bedroom in his house, lifted a can of paint and felt a searing pain in his right shoulder. His shoulder had been a bit sore for the past month, but this pain was like nothing he had ever experienced before. It felt like someone had jabbed an ice pick in his shoulder. He stopped what he was doing, placed a bag of ice on his shoulder, and hoped it would get better. His shoulder improved somewhat in the next few days, but it was still very painful and seemed weaker.

On Monday, he called his primary care physician, Dr. Mark Jeffries. Christopher took the earliest available appointment—seven days later. Dr. Jeffries worked as a solo practitioner in a small office, aided by his long-time office assistant Betty, who scheduled his appointments. He was a friendly and highly efficient doctor. Christopher's visit lasted nine minutes. Dr. Jeffries asked a series of pointed questions about his shoulder symptoms and the injury. Christopher was also hoping to get some advice about his blood pressure. He had noted that it was a bit high when he measured it at the pharmacy the previous week. However, Dr. Jeffries asked Betty to reschedule an appointment for him to discuss his blood pressure in the coming weeks. Dr. Jeffries was concerned that Christopher may have torn the rotator cuff in his shoulder. He ordered an MRI and recommended that he see an orthopaedic shoulder surgeon. He provided Christopher with a list of surgeons but told him that he would need to set up this appointment himself. "I'm sorry, but it can be a bit of a hassle to get an appointment to see these surgeons," Dr. Jeffries said as Christopher was leaving.

That afternoon, Christopher began calling the orthopaedic surgeons. The first three had recorded messages stating they were not presently accepting new patients because their waiting lists were too long. Christopher reached a voicemail on the fourth call, requesting that he call back. On his call to the fifth shoulder surgeon, he was able to reach the surgeon's assistant and scheduled an appointment five months out.

Christopher's symptoms changed considerably in the next five months. His pain, although still present, lessened, but the weakness in his arm seemed to worsen. After a three-month wait, he obtained an MRI that confirmed he had torn part of his rotator cuff.

In early October, five months after his injury, Christopher had his appointment with Dr. Mark Jones. Dr. Jones was an orthopaedic surgeon who was fully certified by the *Royal College of Physicians and Surgeons of Canada*. He specialized in shoulder and knee problems. After his residency training, he had completed a 12-month fellowship in shoulder and knee surgery at a prestigious university teaching hospital. Dr. Jones asked a series of direct questions about the injury. He asked about the treatment Christopher had received to date, as well as his present symptoms. After performing a thorough physical examination, he spent time reviewing the MRI.

Dr. Jones then sat down with Christopher and confirmed that he had in fact suffered a significant tear of his rotator cuff. He explained the implications of this injury. He suggested that while non-operative treatment would likely help his symptoms, because of his relatively young age and the size of the tear, Christopher would benefit from having surgery to repair the rotator cuff tear. Dr. Jones spent some time explaining what was involved in the surgery, including the risks and benefits. He then asked if Christopher would like to proceed with the surgery he had outlined. Christopher said he would.

At that point, Dr. Jones began completing some paperwork. He introduced Christopher to his office assistant Jenny, who would be scheduling the surgery. She apologized that there was quite a wait for surgery and that she did not know exactly when the surgery would be. She estimated that it would be 6 to 8 months from then.

Dr. Jones recommended that Christopher perform some specific shoulder exercises on a regular basis. Christopher began to do these exercises and noted some improvement in his pain and strength. However, he remained symptomatic.

Four months later, Dr. Jones's assistant called, saying they had a surgery date available on March 15—five months after his original appointment with Dr. Jones and almost a year after his initial injury. As the surgery date approached, Jenny gave him some forms to complete, and he was instructed to show up on the morning of surgery without having had anything to eat or drink since midnight. He talked to a representative from the anesthetic team a few days before surgery. They ordered some routine blood tests and an electrocardiogram (EKG), but because of Christopher's relatively young age, he did not require a formal, preoperative medical assessment.

On the day of the surgery, Christopher met Dr. Johnson, the anesthesiologist, for the first time. Dr. Johnson asked a series of questions about previous anesthesia and his general health. He noted that Christopher's blood pressure was a bit high. Christopher said that this had been a bit of an issue over the past year.

The surgery was scheduled for 2:00pm, but at 2:30pm, Dr. Jones came out and apologized that they would need to cancel Christopher's surgery. Apparently, the operating room that Dr. Jones had been assigned only ran until 3:30pm, and his previous surgeries had gone late. Dr. Jones said that on each surgery day, he works with a different team, and for a variety of reasons, today's surgery day had not gone as efficiently as they hoped. Dr. Jones was visibly frustrated with this occurrence. He said his office would reschedule his surgery as soon as possible.

The following week, Jenny from Dr. Jones's office called and said they were able to reschedule Christopher's surgery for May 8—five weeks later. On May 8, Christopher arrived at the preoperative check-in, and the process started again. This time, he was the first surgery of the day, and the surgery went forward uneventfully.

After the operation, he was quite groggy in the recovery room. He vaguely recalled hearing Dr. Jones say the operation went well, but he did not remember any of the details of what was said. Later, when he was more alert, he attempted to clarify some instructions, but Dr. Jones was now back in surgery and the nurse attending to him was not familiar with Dr. Jones' routine. Christopher was discharged home. That evening, he experienced a surprising amount of pain when the anesthetic block wore off. He survived this intensely painful episode and after a few days he started to feel that he was recovering well.

Christopher visited Dr. Jones' office 12 days later and had his sutures removed. Four weeks after surgery, Dr. Jones felt Christopher was doing well enough to start physiotherapy. He wrote a prescription with instructions for Christopher to see a certified physiotherapist. A friend recommended that Christopher see his therapist, and so he scheduled an appointment with Mary Benjamin. He had to pay out-of-pocket for Mary's treatments because physiotherapy treatments performed outside of the hospital were not covered by his provincial medical plan. Mary was enthusiastic and motivated to get Christopher going. She pushed him hard during each therapy session. During one of the sessions two weeks into his therapy, Christopher felt intense pain and heard a pop in his right shoulder while performing a progressive exercise.

Later that week, as part of his regular follow-up, he saw Dr. Jones. He explained the exercise routine that Mary had placed him on; Dr. Jones looked both frustrated and horrified. He calmly but firmly explained that the exercises Christopher was doing were too aggressive. He had been attempting exercises that normally would not be done for another 4-6 weeks. The rotator cuff repair still needed more time to heal and Christopher may have re-ruptured part of the repair in the course of his therapy. Dr. Jones recommended that he back off the therapy and let his symptoms settle.

Christopher's symptoms did settle with less intense therapy, and over time his shoulder improved. Five months after surgery and a year and a half after the initial injury, his shoulder felt okay, but he still had regular pain and felt that his right shoulder was clearly weaker than his left, non-dominant arm. At no point in Christopher's 18-month journey did anyone ask him about his experience or what recommendations he would make to improve the system.

A Traditional Model of Healthcare Delivery in Canada— Contrasted with a Modern, Principle-Based Approach

There are many reasons why someone might seek to visit a doctor within the Canadian health system. The story of Christopher's shoulder injury is just one such example. However, it highlights many elements of the traditional approach to healthcare delivery in Canada. There are many variations on this care delivery system. Based on historical norms and traditional funding models, it represents a stereotypical model of providing medical care. What follows is a contrasting analysis of a traditional model of care delivery within the Canadian system, and a delivery model based on modern principles.

Primary Care: traditional solo practice vs. integrated medical practices

Christopher's experience with his primary care physician highlighted the traditional approach to delivering primary care in Canada. After Christopher aggravated his shoulder, he made an appointment with his primary care physician, Dr. Jeffries, who was in a solo general practice. Dr. Jeffries was compensated on a fee-for-service basis. This meant that each patient visit needed to be fairly quick in order for Dr. Jeffries to make a reasonable income. It also meant that Dr. Jeffries' practice would not have the patient volume or flexibility to easily develop a large-scale, chronic disease management program for common conditions, such as high blood pressure and diabetes. However, at least Christopher had a primary care physician, who could provide some longitudinal care.

Many of his friends resorted to walk-in clinics for their medical care, resulting in expensive, fragmented care with no longitudinal oversight.

Dr. Jeffries' solo practice is contrasted with a modern, team-based approach to providing primary care. Patients still have their own primary care physicians. However, these individuals work as part of a large, multi-disciplined team—such as a *patient-centred medical home* (PCMH)[158]— to provide the needed care. This approach includes preventive care, chronic disease management (diabetes, high blood pressure, etc.), and management of some common specialty conditions (basic orthopaedic and dermatologic problems, etc.). They also have programs to help patients with more complex medical problems navigate the health system (ex. patient navigator programs). By forming a primary care team that includes many non-physician healthcare extenders, who are a less expensive resource to the system than physicians, each team can provide high-quality primary care services to a large group of patients (e.g., 20,000 or more). This type of care is provided at a per-patient cost that is substantially less than a traditional, solo, fee-for-service practice. Such an approach highlights the central role that the delivery of primary care plays in modern healthcare delivery. A good primary care system saves money and lives.

The Relationship Between Primary Care and Specialist Care: a chasm vs. a coordinated interaction

When Dr. Jeffries referred Christopher to an orthopaedic shoulder specialist, he lost oversight of Christopher's shoulder care and left Christopher to deal with the health system on his own. From Dr. Jeffries' point of view, it probably made sense to do this because neither he nor his assistant was compensated for coordinating specialist care. A figurative wall separated primary care and specialist care.

From a diagnostic point of view, Dr. Jeffries ordered an MRI, even though he would not be the physician who would ultimately manage Christopher's shoulder problem. This particular MRI was warranted,

---

[158] *Patient-centred medical homes* may also be referred to as *primary care medical homes.*

although it was not the specific views or settings that Dr. Jones would have ordered. However, many of the MRIs ordered by physicians, who are not ultimately overseeing the patient's care, are unnecessary.[159,160,161] This increases the expense to the system and the wait time for MRIs.

The individual orthopaedic specialists that Christopher tried to obtain a consult with each ran their own practice the way they saw fit. In the traditional healthcare system, they function as individual businesspeople. There was no integration between their practices and their respective waitlists. Furthermore, there was no transparency to their waitlists; neither the time it took to get a consultation (Wait time #1), nor the time from consultation to surgery (Wait time #2) was known. It was unclear whether their long waitlists were real or artificial. An *artificial* or *inflated* waitlist occurs when a specialist consciously sees considerably fewer new patients each week than he or she is capable of, with the unspoken goal of building up a long waitlist. This practice may occur when specialists wants to increase the demand for their services in the private market place; when they decide to spend work time doing other activities that may be more rewarding; or when it is advantageous to build up a long waitlist to obtain some of the political clout that goes with high demand for their services.

Finally, an initial, thorough shoulder assessment did not necessarily require seeing an orthopaedic surgeon. An appropriately trained healthcare extender working in a coordinated manner with an orthopaedic surgeon could render an accurate diagnosis and develop a treatment plan for most common musculoskeletal problems—including shoulder problems.

---

[159] Tocci SL, Madom IA, Bradley MP, Langer PR, DiGiovanni CW. The diagnostic value of MRI in foot and ankle surgery. Foot Ankle Int. 2007 Feb;28(2): 166-8.

[160] Busse J et al. Appropriateness of Spinal Imaging Use in Canada. CIHR sponsored report. April 25th 2013: http://nationalpaincentre.mcmaster.ca/documents/AppropriatenessofSpinalImagingFinalReportApril252013.pdf (accessed December 27th 2015)

[161] http://www.car.ca/files/CAR_Choosing_Wisely_Canada_List_Draft.pdf (Accessed December 27th 2015)

In a modern healthcare system, the primary care physician and his or her team never lose oversight of the patient. Specialists, or more accurately specialty service lines (or teams), are there to help manage more complex aspects of a patient's care, such as Christopher's shoulder injury, but the primary care team helps facilitate this care.

Patients with specific problems may be referred, within the primary care group, to healthcare providers who have a particular expertise (e.g., MSK, endocrine), prior to seeing a specialist. Additionally, for many complex, clinical problems, specialists from the relevant, respective disciplines may be asked into the primary care setting to review prescreened patients in their area of expertise. Also, in a modern system, there will be complete transparency and accuracy of all specialist's wait times (both Wait time #1 and Wait time #2). These steps help ensure that patients will have a minimal wait before an expert sees them.

Episodes of Acute Medical Care: fragmented silos vs. team-based service lines

The entire treatment of Christopher's shoulder problem, including the surgery and recovery, represented a single *episode of care* (EOC), also known as a *care cycle*. His EOC included all of the events related to his shoulder surgery, from the time of the operation until his recovery was complete five months later. EOCs can be identified for almost any medical problem; an EOC can be a single visit to a primary care physician's office for an isolated, self-limiting problem, such as a common cold, or it can include anything that occurs around any prolonged medical or surgical issue—such as treatment for a specific cancer, treatment including hospitalization for a severe medical issue, or the long-term management of a complex, chronic condition, such as renal dialysis.

From a patient-management point of view, an EOC should be viewed as a single entity. However, the traditional Canadian healthcare system presently treats the various events that make up the EOC in isolation—both from a funding point of view and often from a care-coordination point of view.

The cancelation of Christopher's initial surgery date was caused by a lack of coordination and associated inefficiency between the individual members of the surgical team, leading to prolonged surgeries and excessive delays between surgical cases. Without a dedicated shoulder surgery (or musculoskeletal) operating room team, this day was likely the first time in many months (or possibly ever) that Dr. Jones had worked with this particular anesthesiologist and combination of operating room nurses. In the traditional system, the only interaction that the nurses and anesthesiologist would have with Christopher would be on the day of his surgery. As such, they were both beholden primarily to the goals of their respective nursing and anesthesia departments, more than to the final results of the patient's EOC. Unless there was a catastrophic complication, the nurses and anesthesiologists would never receive any feedback on how patients like Christopher did following the surgery. Furthermore, they would not have any formal opportunities to give feedback to the surgeons or other providers involved to improve the overall results—they were completely disconnected from the end results of the EOC.

Mary Benjamin, the physical therapist working on Christopher's shoulder during his recovery, worked in similar isolation. From a surgical point of view, she was practically disconnected from what had previously happened to Christopher. She would have received a short, written physiotherapy order from Dr. Jones, but clearly there had been a miscommunication as to the extent of postoperative therapy that was required.

This type of fragmentation of the EOC is problematic, but it is the norm within the Canadian healthcare system. Without a team-based approach, physicians like Dr. Jones, who witnessed the entire EOC, could not easily convey to everyone involved how their actions affected their patients' overall results. Equally important, the individual healthcare providers could not easily provide feedback to Dr. Jones when they identified an issue that could have improved the overall results for his patients.

Modern healthcare systems organize EOCs around *service lines*— specific teams of multidisciplinary providers, whose mission is to take care of a certain type of clinical problem under the leadership of a single provider. For example, a shoulder service line would likely be made up of orthopaedic surgeons, anesthesiologists, operating nurses, ward nurses, and physical therapists—whose primary job would be to ensure that the shoulder service line functioned effectively.

Those running a modern healthcare system would ensure that service lines were established for any common condition. Each service line would be funded directly, based on quality and productivity. The members of the service line would receive a contracted salary, plus a performance bonus if they qualified. If the service line performed poorly, relative to other equivalent service lines, it would lose its funding and be dissolved. Continued funding is entirely dependent on performance. This approach blows up the traditional department structure, which would no longer need to exist in its traditional form.

Healthcare Funding and Organization: paying for inputs vs. paying for outputs

Christopher's primary care physician, Dr. Jeffries, and his orthopaedic surgeon, Dr. Jones, each got paid on a fee-for-service basis. This money comes directly from the Ministry of Health when physicians submit the appropriate billing claims electronically. These fee-for-service payments directly or indirectly effect how they will run their practices.

Dr. Jeffries sees patients expeditiously, in order to generate a satisfactory income. To do this, he actively discourages addressing multiple complaints during one visit. He is unable to afford hiring additional staff, who could run other programs and help provide care to more patients—because these staff would not be able to bill for their services.

Dr. Jones gets paid for each surgery he performs, which would partially explain his visible frustration when he was forced to cancel Christopher's initial surgery. That decision would have taken $425 out of his pocket, probably through no fault of his own.[162] Furthermore, Dr. Jones may have determined that it was more lucrative for him to use his time in other ways, such as completing medical legal reports,

---

[162] 2013 BC Medical Services Plan Fee code 52505 (Rotator Cuff Repair, simple) pays $425.78. http://www.health.gov.bc.ca/msp/infoprac/physbilling/payschedule/pdf/27-orthopaedics.pdf

performing worker's compensation exams, or seeing patients in a private clinic. In some instances, surgeons have seen the advantages of having a long waitlist, as they know some patients will request to see them at their private practice. Although this is technically illegal, it persists and offers them significantly increased compensation for each patient seen.

The nurses in the operating room and on the recovery ward get paid on an hourly basis. This is the opposite of fee-for-service payments. They will get paid, regardless of how much work is done. In fact, efficiency in this payment model is a negative incentive. If nurses work hard and complete their work efficiently, they are likely to be given *more* work—another surgery to attend or another patient to take care of on the ward.

The flow of money dictates how a health system is organized. In the traditional Canadian system, fee-for-service payments go directly to individual physicians. There is no easy mechanism for physicians to fund healthcare extenders and other employees that they could build a team around—except out of their own billings. The fee-for-service funding mechanism actively disincentivizes organizing large groups to provide coordinated, comprehensive care around their area of expertise. This means that physicians will usually practice solo or in small groups.

This is in contrast with the large, annual, bulk-funding grants each hospital receives. Hospitals receive these yearly grants, largely irrespective of performance. This funding is designed to cover the salary of nurses, administrators, and other hospital employees, essentially dictating that anything beyond routine care needs to be performed, directly or indirectly, via hospital funding. This stifles innovation, as there is a clear tendency to keep the same funding channels open year after year. Additionally, it prevents many surgical procedures and medical treatments from being moved to an outpatient setting, where they could be performed much more efficiently at a significantly lower cost.

Funding and organization of a modern healthcare system is very different. It is organized around three key coordinated elements:

1) team-based primary care programs (e.g., primary care medical homes), whose responsibility is to deliver primary care to its members;

2) service lines, programs, or teams that provide comprehensive management of more complex conditions; and

3) hospitals, surgical centres, or freestanding clinics, who will compete for patients who require use of their facilities.

Funding for each of these groups will be based on bundled payments for care. They will receive a set dollar amount for providing all aspects of care for a certain clinical problem. For example, those running a shoulder service line might receive $9,000 to cover every aspect of a patient like Christopher's care, from the date of surgery until 90 days post-surgery. This payment would come with specific requirements for quality and patient satisfaction. Similarly, hospitals will no longer receive bulk yearly funding as their primary means of financing. Rather, they will receive payments based on the care they actually provide.

With groups such as primary-care medical homes, service lines, and hospitals, each is now expected to deliver clearly specified and understood services. Physicians and other healthcare workers will be hired—either on salary or on a contracted basis—to provide specific services designed to help their respective group achieve its goals. These groups would be examples of the *Integrated Practice Units* (IPUs) that Michael Porter refers to. For example, Dr. Jones might be hired by a shoulder program to work four days per week as part of their team. For two days he would be assigned to work in clinic where he would be expected to see an average of 20 patients per day (including 10 new patients and follow-up assessments on those he had operated on). On the remaining two days he would be assigned to working the operating room performing surgeries on his patients. For this, he would be provided a salary with a productivity bonus.

Being a *team player* would be an essential element for anyone working within this new system—particularly physicians. Failure to perform up to expectations would mean a physician or other healthcare worker would soon find themselves out of a job.

Oversight of the Entire System: an absentee landlord vs. an active system manager

Christopher Barclay is not alone. He is not the only person in his city, his province, or his country with a shoulder problem. There are many other patients like him, just as there are many other patients with other specific medical and surgical problems. Who takes responsibility for ensuring that they have the medical care that they need? Who oversees the system—not just in general terms but in very specific terms? For example, who is responsible for ensuring that the patients in a specific region with shoulder problems get the necessary care? The answer within the Canadian healthcare system is usually *nobody.* A lack of oversight or a *laissez-faire* method to ensuring that populations get the care they need is the traditional approach.

Modern healthcare systems actively coordinate care, not just for specific patients, but for the population as a whole. They practice *population-based healthcare.*[163] They study demographics and trends and predict, with a high degree of accuracy, the type and extent of care that they will need to provide to a specific population—whether it be a city, a health region, or a province. This programmatic approach is essential because physicians, nurses, and most administrators react only to the specific patient-care issues that are directly in front of them. They are not looking at the big picture. That is the responsibility of those individuals who are charged with running the system.

---

[163] The American Medical Association defines population-based medicine as an approach that "allows one to assess the health status and health needs of a target population, implement and evaluate interventions that are designed to improve the health of that population, and efficiently and effectively provide care for members of that population in a way that is consistent with the community's cultural, policy, and health resource values." http://c.ymcdn.com/sites/www.acpm.org/resource/resmgr/policyissues-files/physlicensure_resolution.pdf (Accessed May 2, 2015.)

Traditional vs. 21ˢᵗ Century Healthcare System

There are many manifestations of the traditional Canadian healthcare system, including some segments that deliver excellent care. However, most instances of success occur either because of the determination and excellence of individual healthcare actors, or through finding the means to skirt around traditional, organizational structures. For the bulk of the Canadian healthcare system, historical ways of organizing and funding the system have persisted, making fundamental reform prohibitively difficult (Figure 1).

Figure 1: Traditional Healthcare System: Generic Model

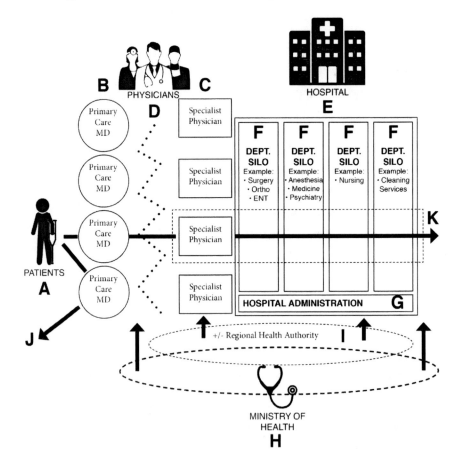

A = Patients

B & C = Primary Care MDs (B) & Specialist MDs (C) paid via fee-for service.

D = Referral wall between primary care MDs and specialist MDs.

E = Hospitals: Primary funding of healthcare is via hospitals and therefore most specialist care is directly or indirectly hospital-based.

F = Siloed departments within hospitals –more closely oriented to their department members than to the patient's episode of care (EOC).

G = Hospital administrators who oversee/control hospital care despite being disconnected from the sites where care is actually delivered.

H = Health Ministry: Governing body? partially oversees healthcare system.

I = Regional Health Authority: Governing body? partially oversees healthcare system.

J = Basic episode of care (EOC): managed by primary care MD (if patient has a primary care MD).

K = Complex episode of care (EOC): Not primary focus of healthcare system. Results of EOC rarely assessed in an accurate manner.

A 21st century healthcare system is highlighted by a more integrated and coordinated way to provide patient care (Figure 2). There is a single governing body that takes ultimate responsibility for the system's performance and actively oversees the system itself. In addition to the governing body, other central elements of the system include three variants of the Integrated Practice Units (IPU) described by Porter:

1) Groups, such as PCMH, that deliver team-based primary care
2) Programs, service lines, or teams that treat specific conditions throughout the entire EOC
3) Hospitals and related healthcare facilities, which interact with the other IPUs to ensure patient care that requires hospitalization is high-quality and cost-effective

Individual actors within the system include doctors, other healthcare providers, administrators, and patients—whose care experience is at the heart of the system.

Figure 2: 21st Century Healthcare System: Generic Model

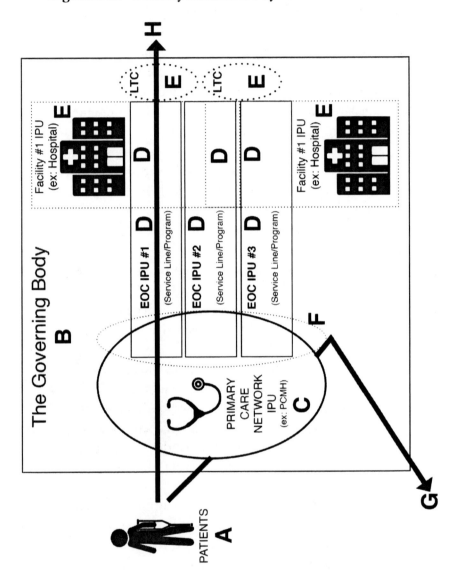

A = Patients: The central focus of a modern healthcare system.

B = The Governing Body. A single governing body that organizes, funds, and is ultimately responsible for all aspects of care the system provides.

C = Patient-centered (or Primary care) Medical Home (PCMH) Integrated Practice Units (IPUs): A groups of healthcare providers (physicians, and healthcare extenders) who work in a coordinated manner to provide primary care to a large group of patients. 90-95% of health care in a modern system is delivered via a PCMH including oversight of LTC.

D = Service Line/Program IPUs: These IPUs coordinate complex episodes of care (EOC). They are made up of physicians, other healthcare providers, and clinically active administrators who are responsible for the results of care.

E = Facility IPUs, including Long Term Care (LTC) IPUs: These IPUs ensure the facilities (hospitals, surgical centres, long term care facilities, etc) are functioning efficiently and safely. They are contracted by service line/program IPUs on a competitive basis.

F = Seamless coordination between primary care delivery and specialized Episodes of Care.

G = Basic episode of care (EOC): PCMH manage 90-95% of clinical problems in a modern healthcare system. Independently collected outcome metrics ensure care is of a high standard.

H = Complex episode of care (EOC): Managed by a by a service line/ program IPU in a coordinated manner. The results of each EOC are assessed by an independent team on a continual basis.

The system is organized so that it can be true to the four core pillars that have been identified:

1) Have clear goals.
2) Create patient-centred teams to achieve goals.
3) Accurately measure the results of care.
4) Pay for outputs, not inputs.

In addition, a series of other principles should guide the actions and functions of 1) those governing the system, 2) teams that function within the system, and 3) physicians and other individual actors working within the system. A modern healthcare system can take many forms. However, to be effective, it will need to adhere to these additional principles, which will be outlined in the next chapter.

Summary: Chapter 7

The three-game Stanley Cup championship series between the Toronto Hockey Club and the Victoria Aristocrats in 1914 had a strong fan base, drawing a total of 14,260 fans to the Toronto Arena—almost 5,000 in attendance per game. However, the 1914 series bore little resemblance to the speed, finesse, and excitement of the Stanley Cup finals one hundred years later. In 2014, each of the five games easily sold out their respective 18,000+ seat arenas, with millions more watching at home on their televisions.[164]

Relative to the hockey played one hundred years later, play in 1914 was pedestrian, poorly coordinated, and unskilled. This quantum leap in performance was the direct product of the way the NHL and the individual teams had come to be organized. The structure of the league had evolved to foster excellence in an evolutionary manner over the previous century; teams that do not function at a high level are quickly exposed. Unfortunately, the structure of healthcare in Canada is more akin to hockey in 1914 than it is to the 2014 version.

Critical to the success of professional hockey has been the central role of the NHL in taking ownership of the game itself. The unspoken mission of the NHL's Board of Directors and Commissioner Gary Bettman is to take every step necessary for the betterment of the game as a whole. Those leading the NHL have understood that the higher the quality, and the more exciting the game of hockey, the more fans watch. The goals of the league, as a whole, trump those of the individual teams. Team owners came to realize that their teams would do better if the

---

[164] Games 1, 2, and 5 were played at the Staples Center in Los Angeles, which has a capacity of 18,118. Games 3 and 4 were played at Madison Square Garden, which has a capacity of 18,006.

league as a whole did better. A solid league foundation that promoted fairness, safety, and excitement was established. Teams came to realize that to do well, they would need to function in a coordinated and skilled manner. Similarly, players knew the rules and quickly came to realize that their individual success would ultimately be tied to the success of their team.

A good, modern healthcare system would be organized in a similar manner to the modern-day NHL. The governing body functions like the NHL: dictating what is best for the system as a whole and ensuring that the best interests of the patients and payers are being served. Just as with the NHL, the goals of the governing body must supersede the goals of specific teams and individual players. Overseen by an individual coach, games are akin to a specific EOC. To win a game, coordinated teamwork is critical. A season is equivalent to multiple, similar EOCs; therefore, a hockey team is equivalent to a service line or IPU. To be successful as a hockey team or a healthcare service line, managers must ensure that all personnel on the team are oriented toward the same goals and are working at full capacity. Similarly, healthcare providers and personnel must be primarily oriented toward the overall goals of their team.

The existing Canadian healthcare system has this organizational structure reversed, which is a product of the system's history. Individual *players* (i.e., physicians) are wildly independent and *play* in a manner that suits their own goals. Teams organized along the lines of the EOC do not really exist, or if they do, they are only loose affiliations. Rather, the primary organizational structure is along departmental lines. This is akin to having all of the goalies in the league being more closely aligned with the other goalies in the league than they are to their own *team*, similarly for defensemen, centres, etc. Finally, the governing bodies (Health Ministries and Health Authorities), unlike the NHL leadership, are weak and ineffectual in ensuring that their constituents (patients and taxpayers) receive the services they require. The end result is a Canadian healthcare system that organizationally has much more in common with professional hockey in 1914, not 2014.

Summary Points: Chapter 7

The flow of money dictates how a health system is organized—and how a system is organized has a direct impact on how it functions.

The Canadian healthcare system funds physicians in isolation from other aspects of the health system, making integrated team-based care delivery difficult or impossible.

Effective modern healthcare systems have a single governing body that actively oversees the system and takes ultimate responsibility for the system's performance.

Modern healthcare systems are funded and organized in a manner that emphasizes three key coordinated elements:

1) Team-based primary care programs whose responsibility is to deliver comprehensive primary care to all patients within the system.
2) Service lines, programs, or teams that provide comprehensive management of more complex conditions.
3) Hospitals, surgical centres, or freestanding clinics that will compete for patients who require use of their facilities.

In addition, modern healthcare systems actively coordinate care, not just for specific patients, but for the population as a whole. They practice *population-based healthcare*, allowing the type and extent of care that they will need to provide to a specific population to be predicted with a high degree of accuracy.

CHAPTER 8

Principles for Running a 21ˢᵗ Century Healthcare System in Canada

The primary goal of the president and the executives of the National Hockey League is to promote the success of the league as a whole. This overarching goal trumps the specific goals of individual teams. Overall success for the league, both on and off the ice, will invariably lead to improved team success. Perhaps this will not produce success in the win column, but it will in terms of increased fan support and financial success. A rising tide raises all ships.

To facilitate success, the league follows some basic principles. These include setting clear goals, using data to drive their decision-making, and penalizing behaviors that undermine their goals.

Similarly, while league goals trump the goals of individual teams, the goals of individual teams trump those of individual players. Decisions are made at the team level, based on what the team's president and general manager believe will ultimately lead to team success. They have a series of principles that they know they will have to adhere to, in order to have a chance for team success.

Individual players bring their specific talents to the game, but they all realize they will be judged in large part by their role in bringing success to their respective teams. There are well-established, basic principles that players recognize they must follow if they are to have individual success playing in the NHL.

The Foot and Ankle Clinic

Prior to my arrival, the British Columbia hospital where I served as department head had instituted an innovative clinic to facilitate the care of patients with foot and ankle problems. The impetus for this program was the excessively long wait times to see one of the hospital's three orthopaedic foot and ankle surgeons. Patients referred by their primary care physicians were waiting six months or more just to be seen by a specialist.

In an effort to address this problem, a group of four primary care doctors were trained to assess, diagnose, and render non-operative treatment to patients with foot problems. These *screening doctors* each worked in the clinic one or two half-days per week. The orthopaedic surgeons trained them, and the idea was for the screening doctors to work beside the surgeons to expedite care delivery in the foot and ankle clinic. Regarding patients whom they had questions about, the surgeons would be on hand to provide guidance. Patients that the screening doctors felt needed a surgical consult would then be referred on for an assessment by one of the orthopaedic foot and ankle surgeons. This approach allowed the hospital's clinic to essentially triple the number of new patients it saw each week.

After an initial startup period during which the screening physicians were trained, the program was instituted and seemed to be quite effective in decreasing the waitlist (Wait time #1) for foot and ankle patients. The clinic was even written up in one of the national newspapers. Within a few months, the waitlist for patients to see a foot specialist was reduced to 4-6 weeks. Furthermore, the patients that were prescreened by the primary care doctors—and were then deemed as requiring a surgical consultation—ended up having an almost 70% chance of requiring surgery, once they did see one of the surgeons.

Subsequently, two problems emerged regarding this program. First, the screening doctors were rarely assigned clinic space that was in close proximity to the orthopaedic surgeons. Therefore they had limited interactions with the specialists when they were in clinic. Everyone got along well, but the surgeons and screening doctors rarely interacted, so mentoring and ongoing teaching was difficult. The second issue was that the surgeon's waitlist did not decrease, and it continued to be highly variable between surgeons. The prescreened patients that were deemed in need of a surgical consult received no expedited care. They were basically placed on the same list that they would have been on if they had been referred directly to the surgeon's office. As it was organized, there was no real benefit to those patients requiring foot surgery.

The solutions to these issues seemed obvious and fairly straightforward. First, ensure the screening physicians worked in a clinic space directly adjacent to the orthopaedic surgeons. This would have allowed for close collaboration between the screening physicians and the surgeons, thereby improving the learning curves of the screening physicians. Second, to address the wait time for orthopaedic surgery consultations, it would seem prudent to expedite the referrals that the screening doctors had seen and decided would potentially need surgical treatment. After all, these patients had a high likelihood of benefiting from a surgical consultation.

These were not the choices made by the administrators who ran the hospital's surgical program, which included oversight of the foot and ankle clinic. Instead, they cut the number of clinics that the screening doctors were running, in an effort to decrease the number of patients they saw. By extension, they decreased the number of patients that were referred on for surgical consultation. Administrators did not view this issue from the perspective of the larger population of patients that needed to be seen. Rather, they were responding to local goals, in this case decreasing an expanding surgical waitlist (Wait time #2) that reflected poorly on their hospital's performance.

This situation was akin to players (administrators and surgeons) being allowed to put their individual goals ahead of the team (the foot service) because there was no overarching mandate from the league's head office (those governing the healthcare system). This type of scenario—whereby individual administrators, physicians, and others involved in the healthcare system made what were, from their perspective, logical decisions that ultimately undermined the whole system—was a recurring feature of the Canadian healthcare system I witnessed. Basic principles of modern healthcare delivery were regularly violated because of the way the system was organized.

This chapter outlines a series of principles that need to be invoked in order to deliver high-value 21st century healthcare, and it reviews an organizational framework for thinking about principle-based care delivery.

Models of Healthcare Delivery: Elements of a Healthcare System

Chapter 7 identified a general model of healthcare delivery that represents the traditional approach (Figure 1), which still predominates within the Canadian medical system. This was contrasted with a general model, illustrating a 21st century, systematized medical system (Figure 2), based on ideas derived from recognized thought leaders described in Chapter 6.

The general model of a 21st century healthcare system is characterized by three important elements: 1) the governing body, 2) three distinct types of teams or *integrated practice units* (IPUs), and 3) three broad groups of individuals functioning within a health system. Continuing the NHL analogy, these elements correspond to: 1) the league head office, 2) the individual teams, and 3) the individual players and personnel.

In the traditional Canadian healthcare system, the governing body is often less clearly delineated, as provincial health ministries often share (or abdicate) oversight of the system to regional health authorities or, in some instances, hospitals. In addition, the three IPUs are replaced by less well-defined mechanisms for: 1) providing primary care delivery, 2) episodes of care, and 3) healthcare facilities. Finally, individual healthcare actors, particularly physicians, are regularly allowed and even encouraged to act in their own best interests, irrespective of the larger interests of the healthcare system.

This chapter will review the following elements of a healthcare system:

1. **The Governing Body**

   Who is overseeing and organizing the system as a whole, in order to ensure the population of patients receives the care they require? What goals have they established for the system, and how will they ensure their goals and priorities are implemented? The governing body has both leadership roles (establishing a vision and a clear direction for the system) and management roles (establishing the manner in which the system is actually run). Principles that guide performance of both of these critical roles will be identified and reviewed.

2. Teams/Integrated Practice Units

- **The Primary Care Network IPUs**

  Primary care physicians and their teams can manage more than 90% of medical problems they encounter.[165] How is the health system organized to ensure ALL patients receive high-quality, timely primary care from healthcare providers—who are fairly compensated and satisfied with their jobs—while reducing overall expenses? The primary care IPUs need to fully address this question.

- **Episodes of Care (EOCs) IPUs**

  Much of the remaining 5-10% of medical care involves specific EOCs. The EOC model provides a key framework for viewing care and, by extension, organizing the provision of care to ensure it is delivered with quality and cost-effectiveness. Service line IPUs should manage EOCs.

- **Hospital (or Facility) IPUs**

  Hospitals are deemphasized in a 21st century healthcare system, as the vast majority of care no longer requires hospitalization. However, there is still a need for high-functioning hospitals and healthcare facilities. These institutions will need to interact with primary care providers, EOC IPUs, and other hospitals to facilitate specialized care delivery.

3. Individuals within a Healthcare system

- **Physicians and Other Healthcare Providers**

  In the accepted medical model, patients are assessed by healthcare providers, a diagnosis is made, and a treatment

---

[165] Barnett ML, Song V, Landon BE. "Trends in Physician Referrals in the United States, 1999-2009."*Arch Intern Med.* 2012; 172(2):163-170. http://archinte.jamanetwork.com/article.aspx?articleid=1108675 (Accessed February 14, 2015.)

plan is developed and carried out. Physicians and other healthcare providers have essential roles, including potential leadership roles within this model (as managers of care delivery). Their behaviour, which is often determined by the existing incentive structure, will be instrumental in determining the success or failure of the system as a whole.

- **Patients**
  Patients and their specific medical needs should be at the centre of the medical system, yet too often their perspective is ignored or deemphasized. Patients also have a responsibility to the system—to help themselves and their fellow patients.

There is no specific way in which all of these elements must be arranged; there are many ways a 21st century healthcare system can be successfully organized. However, there are guiding principles that *must* be adhered to, in order to ensure the resulting medical system is successful. These principles have been identified by reviewing the literature on healthcare reform and business management. They are outlined in categories corresponding to the three broad elements of the healthcare system. Keep in mind that many of the principles (e.g., have clear goals) apply to more than one of these healthcare elements. In addition, there must be a general accountability structure: individual healthcare providers must be accountable to their respective teams/ IUPs, which in turn must be accountable to the governing body.

All too often in the traditional Canadian medical system, some or all of these principles are not followed. This is seen in the example of the Foot Clinic at the start of this chapter. The needs of the patients were not central, otherwise this clinic would have been organized very differently. The clinic was not run as a team-based IPU, centred around a foot and ankle service line; rather, it was run as a series of fragmented doctor-patient interactions. Administrative oversight of this clinic was disconnected from what was happening in the clinics where patients were being seen. Finally, the goals of the clinic were not clear—or if they were clear to administrators (e.g., keep the *official* waitlist below a certain level*)*, they were not reflective of the healthcare needs of the population.

Governing Body Principles

This section outlines 15 principles that should guide the functioning of the healthcare system's governing body. The first principle should be self-evident in a publicly-funded, single-payer health system. However, it is explicitly stated because often it is not invoked—a situation that undermines the entire health delivery process. The four pillars of a 21st century healthcare system, identified in Chapter 6 and reviewed in Chapter 7, are listed as principles 2-5. The remaining 10 principles are not meant to be a comprehensive list.

The 15 governing body principles listed below will be reviewed in more depth in this section:

1. *Have a single governing body that actively manages the healthcare system from the patients' (and taxpayers') perspectives.*
2. *Have clear and specific patient and population outcome goals.*
3. *Promote patient-centred teams, NOT individuals.*
4. *Accurately (and independently) measure the results of care.*
5. *Pay for outputs, not inputs.*
6. *Align incentives.*
7. *Primary care should be the foundation of the healthcare system.*
8. *Ensure that care is coordinated across geography.*
9. *Embrace technology that improves efficiency and quality.*
10. *Respect physicians' (collective) autonomy, NOT physician's (individual) autonomy.*
11. *Eliminate "tollbooths" and "too big to fail."*
12. *Be open to change.*
13. *Minimize bureaucracy.*
14. *Promote transparency.*
15. *Keep politics out of healthcare.*

1. Have a single governing body that actively manages the healthcare system from the patients' (and taxpayers') perspectives.

After my return to Canada, it took me a few months to realize there was no real central oversight of the healthcare system. I thought directives—as to what the system needed—would come via the hospital, acting on behalf of the local health authority or the Health Ministry. They did not. If anything, individual hospitals battled the regional health authority, which in turn battled the ministry for funding and control—each protecting their own turf.

The end result was that healthcare actors, particularly physicians, were often allowed to behave according to their own individual agendas. It was a stunning realization for me, especially when I observed the extent to which individuals would pursue their own agendas—often to the detriment of the system as a whole. Failure to coordinate the entirely predictable healthcare needs of a large group of patients, such as those within a health region or province, represented a system failure on the most basic level.

A successful healthcare system needs to start with an organizational structure that makes sense. A single entity, which is held accountable for the health system's performance and has the power to make changes, is needed to achieve the desired goals. This is how I presumed the Canadian system was organized when I arrived.

The reason for the central importance of this principle is simple. Someone needs to look out for the population as a whole –including the rural and underserved components of that population. This is necessary in order to ensure the healthcare system is providing good value. This is known as *population-based healthcare*. Value in healthcare has been defined as outcomes achieved divided by cost spent.[166]

When treating patients directly in front of them, physicians and other healthcare providers act in what they perceive as the best interest of the patient—they will also naturally tend to act in their own best interest. They rarely consider the larger system, particularly in the traditional, fragmented delivery system. For example, consider a patient who presents to a doctor with a one-week history of foot pain and demands an MRI.

---

[166] Porter ME, Teisberg EO. *Redefining health care: creating value-based competition on results.* Boston: Harvard Business School Press, 2006.

It may be easier and quicker for the doctor to fill out a requisition for an MRI and move the patient (and the associated billing) through his office, than to explain that this test is not indicated at this point in time. Many physicians do the right thing and are conscious of resource allocation on a basic level, but the widespread variation in care tells us that many do not.

A strong governing body needs to actively manage the healthcare system so the goals of the patients and taxpayers are put first. This could be the Ministry of Health, specific Health Regions, or another designated organization—but it cannot be more than one of these. Too many chefs will wreck the meal. Once an active governing body has been clearly established, there are leadership and management principles they must follow. These include the remaining principles described in this chapter. In most instances, these principles are straightforward and self-evident; yet all too often, they are not followed, or they are violated.

2. Have clear and specific patient and population outcome goals.

The Vancouver Coastal Health Authority that I worked within oversees approximately one million patients.[167] How many patients in that region will have a shoulder problem that requires a specialist consultation, and possibly surgery, in the next year? How many hip fractures will occur within the region each year, and how will acute care delivery be coordinated to meet the needs of this patient group? How many will require endocrine-related surgery, and how will the health region manage these patients?

There are a finite number of these types of questions. Furthermore, these questions have answers that can be relatively easily obtained, using known demographics and proactive data collection. Potential solutions to these questions are often surprisingly straightforward and cost-effective. However, if these questions do not even get asked, then clear goals for care delivery within a system will not be generated.

A system must understand what specific problems exist, in order to solve them. When it does, then clear goals can be generated, and establishing clear goals is one of the keys to running a successful

---

[167]   http://www.vch.ca/about-us/

organization, including a healthcare system. The driver of a car needs to know his destination, otherwise he will drive around aimlessly. A health system is no different. Yet a lack of clear goals—or extensive activities that were not in pursuit of any of the established goals—was an almost ubiquitous occurrence within the system I observed.

3. Promote patient-centred teams, NOT individuals.

To the outside observer, our clinic looked like a coordinated foot and ankle program. There were four orthopaedic surgeons, whose elective practices were confined to problems related to the foot and ankle. There were three fellows, two orthopaedic residents, and four screening physicians—all of whom helped provide foot and ankle care.

However, on closer examination, there was no foot and ankle program—just four isolated foot and ankle surgeons doing what they each felt was best for themselves and their patients. They saw whichever patients they wanted to see in whatever order they wanted to see them. They operated on whomever they wanted to, often in whatever order they chose. Some chose to have a relatively short waitlist for clinic patients (Wait time #1) and a long wait time for surgeries (Wait time #2), while others chose the reverse. There was no coordination with the needs of the population, even though our institution specifically received extra funding to promote extra care in this area.

This situation was ripe for a programmatic, team-based approach. However, by tradition, the whims of individual physicians trump the larger organizational goals within the Canadian healthcare system. This deference to the wishes of individual healthcare providers—to the detriment of the larger system—precludes the widespread development of effective IPU-type programs, teams, or service lines.

The principle of promoting programs (i.e. teams), not individuals, is derived naturally from the principle of having clear goals for the institution. Once specific goals are established, they will invariably be better achieved through a programmatic approach. However, in Canada, individual physicians and their idiosyncratic agendas usually rule. This is problematic because decisions are made to suit the individual—and not with the goals and wellbeing of the larger healthcare system in mind.

Furthermore, with multiple individuals all acting independently, wide variations in practice standards and metrics will be the norm. Decreasing variation is one of the hallmarks of quality business organizations—and in healthcare, it saves money and improves the quality of care. A team-based programmatic or service-line approach to care delivery, whether it be primary care or highly subspecialized care, is a much more effective way to promote high-value care that is in sync with the healthcare needs of the population.

4. Accurately (and independently) measure the results of care.

In 2010, patients in Alberta faced long waits for hip and knee replacement surgery. How could this problem be addressed when no additional funding for joint replacement surgery was available? At that point, the Alberta Bone and Joint Health Institute (ABJHI), led by the late Dr. Cy Frank, came upon a straightforward solution—accurately measure what all of the surgeons are doing.[168]

By measuring how long each surgeon's patients stayed in hospital after their joint replacements and sharing this data (with the various surgeons' names blinded), each surgeon could see how he or she was doing compared to his or her colleagues. In addition, they promoted the use of standardized clinical care pathways for total knee and hip replacements, encouraged the development of local, multi-disciplinary teams (doctors, nurses, and administrators), and convinced the government to let them reinvest any money that was saved back into providing joint replacement surgeries.

When surgeons saw objective data as to how they were performing relative to their colleagues, they pushed to improve their performance, and—with team support and increased standardization—the results were dramatic. By 2012, the ABJHI program had saved over 13,500 bed-days per year, freed up enough funds to perform more than 1,000 additional joint replacements each year, and were well on their way to reducing wait times for hip and knee replacements to below their goal of 14 weeks.

---

[168] http://umanitoba.ca/outreach/evidencenetwork/archives/4982

To be effective, payments for outputs must be combined with accurate outcome measures. Just like any consumer, it is critical that governing bodies understand what they are actually getting for the money they are paying. How satisfied are patients who received their care from Dr. Y? What is the post-operative infection rate for procedure A at hospital B? How well do patients with condition C do when they are treated at institution D? What is the cost of care for each patient undergoing a specific treatment at hospital E? And as the ABJHI reviewed, what is the average length of stay for hip replacement patients among various surgeons?

These are examples of outcome metrics—and outcome metrics are one of the cornerstones of modern medicine. Outcome measures need to be acquired in at least four broad categories: 1) patient satisfaction, 2) outcomes of treatment, 3) complication rates, and 4) costs per episode of care. How can patients and health administrators make reasonable decisions if they do not know what the existing system is presently delivering?

How can those governing the healthcare system hold individuals accountable for their team or program's performance if they do not know the results they are presently achieving? Accurate outcome measures help facilitate system accountability. Accountability has been defined as having to be answerable to someone for meeting defined objectives.[169] The elements of accountability include specifying what, by whom, to whom, and how.[170] Professional hockey players are accountable to their team and those governing the league, teams are accountable to the league, and those running the league are accountable to team owners –and indirectly to fans. Similarly, in healthcare there are layers of accountability, but ultimately those running the healthcare system must to be held accountable for the systems' performance. To ensure this accountability accurate outcome metrics are essential.

---

[169] Emanuel, EJ, Emanuel LL. What Is Accountability in Health Care? *Annals of Internal Medicine.* 1196, 124(2): 229–39. doi: 10.7326/0003-4819-124-2-199601150-00007.

[170] Deber RB. Thinking about Accountability. *Healthcare Policy.* Vol 10, Special Issue, Sept 2014. http://www.longwoods.com/content/23932 (Accessed February 6th, 2016)

Programs like that at the ABJHI and the National Surgical Quality Improvement Program (NSQIP) demonstrate the benefits of accurate outcome metrics. However, what was striking to me was that, in general, *accurate* outcome metrics were decidedly absent from the healthcare system I observed. This is not to say there were no metrics—quite the opposite. Strategies to assess overall patient satisfaction, complication rates, and cost of care were often present, but usually lacked specificity and accuracy. This prevented the results of these measurements from providing meaningful feedback to existing care delivery. Existing data collection was akin to comparing apples and oranges –all while suspecting the various fruits were probably bad.

The Canadian Institute for Health Information (CIHI) was formed in 1994 to "provide essential information on Canada's health system."[171] CIHI has noble and well-intentioned goals. However, much of the CIHI data is macroscopic, based on nationally-derived, de-identified patient data—thereby providing limited feedback for specific programs.

Data collected by local or regional institutions are at times voluminous, often keeping administrators occupied in their offices for hours at a time. They study their computer screens and are lulled into thinking they have a good understanding of what is happening down on the healthcare playing field. However, most data is either collected in an inaccurate manner or does not represent an important aspect of care delivery. Long stay (ALC) bed-days are often measured inaccurately, complication rates are notoriously underreported and opaque, and patient feedback is either not measured or is too generic to guide overall care delivery.

Outcome metrics must represent an important outcome, and they must accurately reflect what they are intended to measure. To ensure that outcome metrics are accurate, they need to be *independently* measured by those outside of the organization. For example, the governing body of a healthcare system could appoint an independent group to collect outcome metrics for all of the hospitals and physicians within the system. Accurate outcome metrics are exactly what a healthcare system needs,

---

[171] http://www.cihi.ca/CIHI-ext-portal/internet/EN/Theme/about+cihi/
cihi010702

but are not necessarily what physicians and healthcare administrators are looking for. Data that allow direct comparisons among hospitals, programs, and physicians have the very real potential to make their job more difficult.

5. Pay for outputs, not inputs.

"Here is $700 million dollars. We will be back this time next year. Don't spend it all. Oh, but spend most of it; otherwise, we will not give you as much next year." The dollar figures vary by hospital, but in essence, this is how most hospitals in Canada, including the one I worked at, have been funded.

"See as many patients as you would like, as fast as you would like, with whatever level of care and service you would like. We will pay you for each patient you see. The more patients you see, the more money you will make." This is the reality of fee-for-service medicine[172]—still the primary mechanism by which doctors are compensated in Canada.

Hospitals and the care they facilitate are *inputs* to the healthcare system. Isolated physician visits, surgeries, x-rays, and other tests are also *inputs*—fragmented parts of a larger whole. All of these elements may be essential at various points in the patient's episode of care. However, they should not be paid for in isolation from the overall results of care— the *outputs* of the healthcare system. By this definition, an example of an *output* would be a patient with debilitating hip arthritis who was fully recovered from a hip replacement surgery three months after the procedure. The doctors' visits, x-rays, surgery, hospitalization, nursing care, and physiotherapy the patient received would all be considered inputs to the systems. Using this framework the fundamental unit of healthcare delivery is changed to reflect the entirety of care and not the individual parts.

It is fairly straightforward to determine what *outputs* are needed from a healthcare system. The primary care medical needs of specific populations must be addressed; hospitalized acutely ill patients must be effectively

---

[172] This assumes an excess patient demand, as is the norm for most practitioners in Canada. If there were not excessive demand then patients would migrate towards those practitioners who they felt provided the best care.

treated; patients with surgical conditions must have their surgery and the associated post-surgical treatment so a good result is realized; and chronic diseases such as diabetes, heart disease, and high blood pressure must be successfully managed over specific time periods. These are all *outputs*. To obtain a successful output the various inputs to the system must function in an integrated manner as part of the larger whole.

Bundled payments are an effective method of paying for outputs rather than inputs. Specific lump sum payments for the end-result of care force those overseeing the system to focus on the end result of patient care whether it is managing an acute illness or surgery from start to finish, treating the primary care needs of a defined population, or managing a chronic illness or mental health issue for a set period of time. Inherent in this approach is the need to apply some basic risk adjustment to account for differences in patient populations (ex. related to age, socioeconomic status, etc.) and the need to ensure that there is appropriate coordination of long-term care management where applicable. This approach not only rewards, but demands value, innovation, and teamwork. *Bundled payments* create a strong impetus to improve care and efficiency.

However, *paying for outputs* is not the traditional funding model that has been employed in Canada. Instead, the Ministries of Health fund hospitals with yearly bulk payments—also known as *global budgeting*. This funding occurs directly or indirectly via regional health authorities. Bulk payments with no associated *outputs* serve to actively disincentivize improved care. Similarly, fee-for-service physician compensation encourages high-volume, fragmented care that does not focus on the end results. Both *global budgeting of hospitals* and *fee-for-service* funding models cement the status quo and eliminate the incentive to innovate.

6. Align incentives.

Surgeons get paid for each operation they perform. Operating room nurses get paid per hour. The results are that the surgeons want to move efficiently, and the nurses are disincentivized to move quickly. Most surgeons love to operate. However, the frustration among my orthopaedic surgical colleagues was palpable. At least half the surgeons talked to me at some point during my time as department head and told me how frustrating it was to operate at our hospital.

Individuals respond to the incentive structure they are working under, so it is critical that the incentive structure be aligned to foster high-quality, cost-effective healthcare. When physicians are compensated based on the volume of care they provide, rather than the quality, a lot of patients are seen rapidly, but they may not have their specific healthcare needs met. Those governing the system can and should change the incentive structures to foster the type of care that is needed.

7. Primary care should be the foundation of the healthcare system.

While I worked in Canada, I never had a primary care physician. Fortunately, I did not have a problem that demanded medical attention. On three occasions, I attempted to find a primary care physician. It seemed that whenever I called a physician who had been recommended, they were not taking new patients. Without a pressing reason to see a doctor, I gave up; like many of my friends and acquaintances, I did not have an established primary care physician to quarterback my healthcare needs.

Johns Hopkins School of Public Health cites this definition of primary care: *The level of a health services system that provides entry into the system for all new needs and problems, provides person-focused (not disease-oriented) care over time, provides care for all but very uncommon or unusual conditions, and coordinates or integrates care, regardless of where the care is delivered and who provides it. It is the means by which the two main goals of a health services system, optimization and equity of health status, are approached.*[173]

A robust, integrated, outcome-oriented primary care system is at the heart of a good medical system. Focusing on primary care delivery places an emphasis on care that is less expensive and is usually more effective. Regardless of whether a healthcare governing body oversees a community of 10,000 or an entire province, it needs to ensure there is a well-organized primary care program. Effective primary care delivery

---

[173] http://www.jhsph.edu/research/centers-and-institutes/johns-hopkins-primary-care-policy-center/definitions.html

is the foundation of the healthcare system, and it needs to be designed to meet the specific primary care needs of that system.

Approximately 90% of medical conditions can (and should) be managed effectively at the primary care level. The Canadian medical system is positioned to deliver consistently excellent primary care. However, it fails to achieve this basic goal—not because of the lack of skills or effort of the individual practitioners, but because of the way the system itself organizes primary care delivery.

In Canada, many citizens are like I was. They do not have a primary care provider to oversee their healthcare needs. Furthermore, those individuals fortunate enough to have a primary care physician often receive fragmented care that fails to provide effective, longitudinal management of chronic healthcare issues.

The fee-for-service *physician compensation model* promotes a "refer and move on" approach. It also precludes the hiring of healthcare extenders (medical office assistants, physician assistants, and nurses), who—if they worked closely with primary care physicians—could substantially increase the volume and quality of primary care that is provided.[174]

8. Ensure that care is coordinated across geography.

While working on-call as an orthopaedic surgeon at my old job, it was fairly common to get a call from *BC Bedline*[175]—a provincial program that integrated all of the hospitals within the province with respect to urgent medical issues. A typical patient would have suffered a hip fracture or lower leg (tibia) fracture and was presently waiting in the emergency room of an outlying hospital that did not have access

---

[174] In the existing Canadian fee-for-service system, only a physician can bill for seeing a patient. Therefore, a physician assistant—or other healthcare extender working on behalf of a physician—who oversees these individuals' care delivery cannot legally bill for patients that are seen exclusively by a healthcare extender.

[175] Now called the *BC Patient Transfer Network.*
http://www.bcehs.ca/our-services/operating-entities/bc-patient-transfer-network

to orthopaedic care. More serious trauma patients would go to the Regional Trauma Centre.

Whenever I received a call from *BC Bedline*, I would check with the nursing supervisor about bed availability. If we could accept the patient, which we always tried to do, I would then talk to the physician at the referring hospital. A plan would be outlined, often having the patient transferred by ambulance to our hospital. When the patient arrived, they would be admitted to our hospital and prepared for surgery. One of my colleagues or I would perform the needed surgery, and then when they had been stabilized, they would be transferred back to the original hospital.

BC Bedline illustrates an excellent example of how care—in this case, the coordination of acute emergency care—can be successfully coordinated across geography. Unfortunately, this sort of coordination between institutions was the exception, not the norm.

Patients requiring specialist care were usually treated within a vacuum and confined to the hospital that their treating physician was affiliated with. Typically, there was very little interaction or understanding of the day-to-day goings-on of other hospitals, even though they may have only been 5 or 10 km away. This occurred in spite of the fact that we were often treating identical problems in identical patient populations. This is the traditional model of *full-service* hospital care. It is a model that is now outdated.

21st century medicine demands a system that is integrated across geography. This approach allows for a concentration of expertise in regional centers, while less expensive, basic care is performed at outpatient centres or community hospitals. Expanding the geographic reach of high-value healthcare organizations improves the quality of care and decreases the overall cost. It is a concept that a centralized, coordinated healthcare governing body could institute with relative ease.

9. Embrace technology that improves efficiency and quality.

"I don't understand your concerns regarding the clinic's computers. They are only four years old." That was the comment from an administrator on one of the many occasions when my colleagues and I expressed our frustrations with the existing computers and IT system. Digital x-rays were taking an extraordinary long time to load, grinding our clinic flow to a halt. It would have been generous to describe the hospital's electronic medical record (EMR) system as cumbersome. Individual physicians used their own EMRs, which could not communicate with the other EMRs. Sending or faxing a letter was often still the fastest way to get patient information where it needed to be. In an era where computers and IT have transformed society, we were practicing medicine in a technology abyss. The health system was still trapped in the 1990s.

21st century healthcare systems need to embrace technology, but it needs to be done in such a way that both quality and efficiency are improved. Michael Porter emphasizes building an enabling information technology platform as one of his six steps for reforming a healthcare system. Having rapid access to every patient's up-to-date medical record is critical to providing high-quality, efficient care. Clearly, patient confidentiality must be protected. However, it is possible to do this and still ensure that lab tests, consultation notes, and recent x-rays are available to be reviewed by clinicians. A single medical record system or, more practically, a series of systems that can communicate with each other would achieve this goal.

However, implementing a comprehensive EMR system to improve quality cannot be done without a great deal of attention to the effect it will have on workflow. Inputting extensive and often mundane patient information for hours each day—to fulfill the EMR content requirements—is not the best use of physicians' time. Forcing a fundamental workflow change on physicians and other healthcare providers can decrease their efficiency by 30% or more. Such a change will naturally be met with intense resistance by those actually providing patient care.

Any EMR system needs to be designed and implemented by individuals who actually take care of patients, not merely imposed on a system by bureaucrats or IT specialists who are disconnected from how patient care is delivered. However, once fully incorporated, a comprehensive EMR system that is widely used will have a transformative effect on the healthcare system.

10. Respect physicians' (collective) autonomy, NOT physician's (individual) autonomy. (Decreasing variation is a hallmark of quality improvement.)

From Monday through Thursday each week, our hospital clinic hosted four different orthopaedic surgeons—each on a different day. These surgeons had an identical practice population. However, they each took a very different approach to their practice. In clinic, one surgeon would see an average of 18 patients per day, another 25, another 32—and the fourth averaged 50 patients per day. Similarly, there was large variation in their wait times, their indications for surgery, and their complication rates. Throughout Canada, wide variations in practice patterns have been the norm for years. Often these variations were not merely 5-10%, but rather 100-200% or more.[176,177]

A physician's autonomy to practice independently according to their *professional judgment* has traditionally been viewed as a birthright of any board-certified physician. However, this approach violates a fundamental principle that has been validated in every other industry— decreasing variation in a system is a hallmark of improved quality.[178]

To ensure high-quality care, a governing body that organizes and oversees a health system must focus on decreasing variations in practice. To do this requires a movement to establish *best practices* and other tools to promote standardization, such as *care pathways* that have been shown to help minimize variation and improve care. In this model, individual healthcare providers are still expected to render treatment decisions, according to their judgment. However, by establishing treatment norms for all common conditions, by reviewing when (and

---

[176] http://www.dartmouthatlas.org/keyissues/issue.aspx?con=1338 (Accessed May 10, 2015.)

[177] Large variations in healthcare use across provinces and territories in Canada raise questions about the efficiency and equity of health service delivery. http://www.oecd.org/canada/Geographic-Variations-in-Health-Care_Canada.pdf (Accessed December 31st, 2015.)

[178] "What is the Law of Variation?" American Society for Quality website, based on Timothy J. Clark's *Success Through Quality: Support Guide for the Journey to Continuous Improvement*, ASQ Quality Press, 1999.
http://asq.org/learn-about-quality/variation/overview/overview.html (Accessed April 28, 2015.)

why) treatment decisions fall outside of these norms, and by holding individuals accountable for their treatment decisions, a dynamic, high-quality system with decreased practice variation will evolve.

Keys to achieving a decrease in clinical variation are promoting *physicians' collective autonomy* and discouraging individual *physician's autonomy*. It is critical that treatment decisions be made by physicians and healthcare providers, rather than imposed by disconnected administrators. To this end, it is reasonable, and in fact desirable, that a *group* of physicians practicing in the same discipline be asked to work together to develop and agree upon standardizing equipment needs, personnel requirements, and treatment guidelines for common conditions. This is an example of *physicians' autonomy*—allowing a group of physicians to collectively agree how they would like to approach a certain situation.

Ultimately, the results they achieve will be compared to other teams that provide similar or identical services. If the group as a whole underperforms based on outcomes, they will collectively be held accountable. However, promoting physicians' autonomy will not only have the effect of decreasing variation, but also improving quality as individual physicians are challenged to reevaluate how they are practicing—by reviewing the evidence-based literature and engaging in negotiations with their peers.

11. Eliminate "tollbooths" and "too big to fail."

Each June, the department of anesthesia at my hospital would inform the hospital's Surgical Business Committee how many operating room days they would not be able to cover, due to the summer vacation plans of their members. The number of operating room days that needed to be cancelled was often in the hundreds. During those days, the flow of surgical patients ground to a halt.

In the existing Canadian healthcare system, anesthesia is an example of a *tollbooth*. A group that functions as a tollbooth has the ability to shut down a road—in this case a surgical episode of care—despite only intersecting with that *road* in one place. *Tollbooths* are also positioned to extract a heavy fee from the system for use of the road—if they choose to do so.

Anesthesiologists are not the only example of *tollbooths* in the Canadian healthcare system that I witnessed. Any group that intersects with the episode of care at one or more points—and is critical to the success of the patient's treatment but is *not* tied to the ultimate success or failure of the episode of care—is a *tollbooth*. These groups also include radiologists who read imaging studies and laboratory services that evaluate blood tests. Eradicating *tollbooths* is conceptually straightforward -ensure that they are directly tied to the results of the larger episode of care. This is achieved by aligning individuals primarily with specific programs and not their traditional departments.

The hospital I worked at received more than $700 million dollars of budgeted funding each year—most of it from the provincial government. It was *too big to fail*. It will never be closed, nor should it be. Some of the services it provided were outstanding, many were average, and some were poor. However, the funding and management model that was used did not provide a meaningful way to eliminate or dramatically alter poorly performing services. In the existing Canadian system, most hospitals are destined to receive large bulk funding on an annual basis because they are simply too big to fail.

Groups that are *tollbooths* and institutions that are *too big to fail* can, and often do, negatively impact the efficiency and effectiveness of the healthcare system. Their existence highlights the need to reform the healthcare system, in order to eliminate these impediments to care delivery.

12. Be open to change.

My orthopaedic practice, the practices of most of my physician colleagues, and the hospital as a whole would have stopped functioning— or at least would have been significantly interrupted—if all of the fax machines had stopped working. Faxing was still one of the most common ways of exchanging information within the healthcare system at the time.

The fax machine was a revolutionary idea in 1966 when Xerox introduced the Magnafax Telecopier—the first commercially available fax machine. Its popularity as a business tool soared in the 1970s and '80s, before it was overtaken by email and other internet-related ways of more efficiently exchanging information. However, this transition still does not seem to have happened in many parts of the Canadian medical system. Changing a medical system is difficult. Yet fundamental change is exactly what is needed.

All systems are changing, some faster than others. Change is essential in order for systems such as the healthcare system to be able to improve the services they provide. There are two general types of changes: *evolutionary change* and *disruptive change*. A health system needs to be open to the possibility of both types of change. Introducing and managing change can be almost impossible in a large system that is gummed-up by tradition. Such is the situation facing the present Canadian healthcare system. Yet the job of those governing such a system is to make these types of changes possible.

Evolutionary change occurs when the existing process is sound and steady; incremental improvements are made to produce a better and better service, often at a lower cost. Imagine the Postal Service, which started delivering mail via horse and carriage during the 1800s. With the advent of railway lines, the speed of cross-country mail improved. The use of airmail delivery began in 1918, leading to still quicker mail delivery and a wider network. An automated mail sorter was introduced in 1957. Postal codes were instituted in 1971. Advances like these led to the steadily-improving efficiency of the mail system over time. This is an example of evolutionary change. There are many opportunities for these types of changes within every health system. Process improvement tools, such as lean thinking and the use of the Six Sigma strategies, can be used to foster improvement in any existing process.

There are times when a process is rendered outdated by time, or via new discoveries. *Disruptive change* (non-linear innovation) often leads to a dramatically better way of achieving the goals of the system.[179,180] Consider again the delivery of messages between individuals. For over 200 years, since its founding in 1775, Canada Post or its forebears had been the primary means of transmitting written communication. However, with the advent of the internet, the majority of our written communications are now delivered via email. This is an example of *disruptive change.*

There are many examples in the healthcare system where a radical new approach characteristic of *disruptive change* would be profoundly beneficial. This includes a fundamental redesign of the entire healthcare system's organizational structure. Many programs that presently exist within hospitals could be moved to outpatient settings. Technology can be incorporated to improve care via telehealth. The isolated primary care physician can be transitioned to a patient-centred medical home.

Disruptive change in healthcare offers the real potential to dramatically improve patient care and markedly decrease cost. However, *disruptive change* can only occur if those governing the system actively create the opportunity for these types of changes to occur—something that has, as of yet, failed to occur within the Canadian healthcare system in any meaningful way.

---

[179] Disruptive innovation is a business concept described by Clayton Christensen (Bower JL, Christensen CM. Disruptive Technologies: Catching the Wave. *Harvard Business Review* Jan-Feb 1996). In Christensen's outline of disruptive innovation he describes the initial disruption as being "a different package of attributes valued only in emerging markets remote from, and unimportant to, the mainstream." (The Innovator's Dilemma. Boston, MA USA. Harvard Business School Press, 1997). However, the use of the terms *disruptive change* or *non-linear innovation* in the above setting does not imply an inferior service or results.

[180] An alternate definition of disruptive innovation is "the introduction of new technologies, products or services in an effort to promote change and gain advantage over the competition. In this context, the word disruptive does not mean to interrupt or cause disorder—it means to replace." http://searchcio. techtarget.com/definition/disruptive-innovation (Accessed December 30th 2015).

13. Minimize bureaucracy.

As orthopaedic department head, I was a member of 12 hospital committees. Most met monthly, almost always for an hour or longer. The committee members were invariably friendly, and at times funny. Coffee and donuts were regularly served. The meetings were usually boring, but otherwise pleasant. However, we rarely got anything meaningful accomplished. There was a lot of talk, but little action.

The bureaucracy I experienced within the Canadian healthcare system was not confined to committee meetings; it was everywhere. One of the first people an orthopaedic surgeon starting at a new hospital meets is the nurse in charge of coordinating orthopaedics in the operating room. One of the main responsibilities of this person is to ensure that surgeons have the surgical instruments they need. Having a standardized instrument set allows a surgeon to have the equipment he or she requires during each operation.

At the hospitals I had previously worked at in the USA, ordering and obtaining a foot-and-ankle instrument set typically required a pleasant, 10-minute conversation with the nurse in charge of equipment—followed by a two-week wait for the equipment to arrive. In Canada, accomplishing the same thing took over a year and more than 50 hours of my time. The saga of obtaining these instrument sets included multiple one-on-one meetings, countless emails, many committee meetings, and long delays to wait for *order processing*. The reliance on committee meetings and the inefficiency with which committees worked were emblematic of the stifling bureaucracy within the system. The failure of any committee or individual to get anything accomplished without a Herculean effort was devastating to productivity—and morale.

Understandably, there is a certain amount of bureaucracy in any large institution. An example of hospital bureaucracy is the large number of hospital administrators, who are often completely disconnected from what is happening—with respect to the clinical care of patients. Their days seem to be filled with an endless array of meetings. Unwittingly, they function like a glue to jam up the workings of the healthcare system. However, active steps can be taken to manage and limit this bureaucracy.

There is a tendency to think problems are easier to solve when a group of people get together to discuss solutions. The reality is that "the desire to reach consensus and avoid confrontation hinders progress;" this is according to David McRaney in his book *You Are Not So Smart*.[181] When individuals get together in groups of five or more, such as most committee meetings, there is an evolutionary tendency to not want to disagree.

As McRaney points out, *"It turns out, for any plan to work every team needs at least one asshole who doesn't give a shit if he or she gets fired or exiled or excommunicated. For a group to make good decisions they must allow dissent and convince everyone they are free to speak their mind without risk of punishment."* This is not what happens in most situations where committees meet. It is certainly not what I observed; on the contrary, everyone was excessively nice. Unfortunately, being agreeable and nice in this setting predictably leads to higher costs, less care delivered, higher complication rates, and more patient deaths. As a result, groups of greater than five people will regularly make poor decisions—often reaching a false consensus to persist with the status quo, when clear change is warranted.

More than wasting valuable human resources, bureaucracy crushes the spirit of an institution. When individuals working within a system see that it is not possible to get things done or enact needed changes, they eventually give up trying. The governing body of a health system needs to be constantly on the lookout for ways to minimize bureaucracy. Every effort must be made to reshape and reorganize the system to ensure things can get done and that needed changes can be implemented. Bureaucracy is the silent killer of the healthcare system.

14. *Promote transparency.*

Financial and organizational transparency is critical to successfully running a healthcare organization. Financial transparency is essential because huge cost savings can be identified when more individuals within the system have an understanding of various costs, and how

---

[181] *You Are Not So Smart.* David McRaney. Chapter 23 (*Groupthink*). Published by Penguin Group (USA), Inc. New York, NY. 2011.

money is being spent. Organizational transparency is important because people need to know what each person's role and responsibility are within the system. Who is responsible for the various tasks that need to be done? When specific individuals are responsible for performing certain activities, it is easier to determine who to talk to when those activities do not get performed—or get performed at a substandard level. All too often in the existing system, no one is responsible. Problems are blamed on the amorphous system, with no real possibility for change.

15. Keep politics out of healthcare.

My first exposure to politics in healthcare came during my residency. A high- profile politician had a relatively minor injury. Because of political pressure, the orthopaedic service was forced to perform his surgery ahead of far more urgent patients. This sort of queue-jumping is now the norm—and not just for politicians, but for high-level administrators, physicians, and well-connected citizens.

However, cutting to the front of the healthcare line is relatively innocuous compared to some of the other political maneuvering surrounding healthcare. Infrastructure funding to build or renovate hospitals often seems to be based more on political pressure than on need. Costly programs and outdated practice models continue to be promoted because political pressure often precludes more reasoned decision-making.

Given the existing funding and organizational structure, it is presently not possible to keep politics entirely out of the healthcare system. This is one of the primary arguments for fundamental system reform. Decisions regarding the healthcare system should be based on solid principles, not politics. Similarly, medical decisions should be based on what is best for the patient, not what politicians will or will not allow.

What self-interested communities or individuals want from the healthcare system is often not in the best interest of the healthcare system as a whole. Yet by working through their local politicians, individuals and communities can often force through their agenda.

Catering to special interest groups is not only expensive, it often leads to bad medical care and potentially undermines the entire system.

If delivering high-value care is the primary goal of the healthcare system, then *management* of the system needs to be kept at arm's length from the politicians. Conversely, as the elected representatives of the people, politicians should set goals for the healthcare system, assess whether these goals have been met, and hold those running the system accountable for the results achieved.

Governing Body Principles: Summary

The NHL head office makes decisions on behalf of, and for the good of, the league as a whole—with powers that trump both the wishes of individual teams and individual players. 21st century healthcare delivery dictates that within each health system, the governing body overseeing and bearing responsibility for care delivery needs to function in a similar manner. In Canada, this organization (whether it be a provincial health ministry or a regional health authority) must primarily represent the people their health system services—the patients who are treated and taxpayers who fund it.

The principles that have been presented here are intended to be self-evident—naturally-derived from the structure of 21st century team-based healthcare delivery. These principles are not all-inclusive, nor do they dictate a narrow manner within which a good healthcare system needs to be run. There can be many different manifestations of high-value healthcare systems that still adhere to these ideas. However, a failure to incorporate these principles will seriously undermine the effectiveness of a health system—a reality that has been illustrated within most manifestations of the existing Canadian healthcare system.

Integrated Practice Units (Healthcare Teams): Guiding Principles

While the NHL head office organizes and oversees the sport, individual teams play the actual games. Similarly, in 21st century healthcare, the governing body must provide the organizing structure and define the broad system goals, but teams need to deliver the actual care. This section reviews the principles that will help ensure the healthcare team that is actually delivering the care is functioning effectively.

The individual physician was preeminent in 20th century medicine. However, 21st century medicine demands a fundamental paradigm shift to address the increasing complexity of care provision. To achieve this goal requires a systematized, team-based approach.

There are three broad categories of healthcare teams: 1) primary care teams, 2) specialty service line teams, and 3) facility (e.g., hospital) teams. There are clear principles that need to guide the functioning of each of these teams. These principles are derived from experiences in other industries, as well as the ideas that underpin modern healthcare delivery. Failure to adhere to these principles will undermine the quality of care that the system delivers and/or increase the cost of care.

In defining a 21st century healthcare team, a variation of Michael Porter's definition of an *Integrated Practice Unit (IPU)* will be used:[182] An IPU is a type of program in which a series of coordinated individuals and events work together to achieve a common goal, whether it is to provide primary care services to a population over a set period of time, provide the full cycle of care to patients with a certain condition, or run a facility in a highly-functional manner so other teams may deliver care in that venue. A healthcare team may also be referred to as a *service line*—a group of coordinated individuals and resources that work together to deliver a specific service. Therefore, the terms *IPU, program,* and *service line*—while not identical—will be used to describe various modern, coordinated healthcare teams.

The goal for these teams (except facility teams) is to deliver a successful *episode of care* (EOC) to each patient they treat. To accommodate for the fact that many conditions extend over a long period of time, a time component is often added to the EOC definition. A single EOC is to the healthcare team what a hockey game is to a hockey team, and multiple EOCs performed by the same healthcare team over a set period of time is analogous to a hockey season.

---

[182] Porter ME, Lee TH. The Big Idea: *The Strategy That Will Fix Health Care.* The Harvard Business Review Oct 2013. P.53

How realistic is it to segment care when every patient is different? Yes, it is true that every patient is different—and a healthcare system needs to accommodate these differences. However, this is also true for hockey—no two games are ever exactly the same. Yet each game is the same on a basic level. The length of each game is the same. The rules of the game are the same. And the qualities that are likely to lead to success in each game are the same. This commonality allows those leading a hockey team to prepare for each game, and the season as a whole, in a manner that will optimize their chance for success. Healthcare teams need to employ a similar approach.

To ensure teams are delivering high-value patient care, a principle-based approach is required. The following 12 principles for running an integrated practice unit (healthcare team) are outlined in this section:

1. *Actively strive for truly patient-centred care.*
2. *Teams must be formed around the episode of care (EOC).*
3. *Programs should focus on addressing clear goals, which need to be established by the health system.*
4. *Strong program leadership, which is responsible for the entire EOC, is essential.*
5. *A culture of excellence must be fostered among the entire team.*
6. *Individual team members need to be held accountable for their performance.*
7. *Outcomes must be independently measured.*
8. *Quality improvement initiatives should be incorporated into every program.*
9. *Healthcare providers should practice to the limits of their licenses.*
10. *Primary care delivery programs should be multidisciplinary, coordinated, and outcome-oriented.*
11. *Compensation should be aligned to promote high-value care.*
12. *Programs that underperform should be reformed or eliminated.*

1. Actively strive for truly patient-centred care.

There is an unwritten rule in medicine. Any patient who tells you they have a *high pain threshold* invariably does not. Patients who actually have a high pain tolerance suffer stoically. When asked if they are in discomfort after a major pain- invoking event, they will say something like, "Yep, Doc, this is a tough one."

Providing *patient-centred care* is somewhat akin to pain tolerance. Those organizations that tell you they are providing *patient-centred care* usually are not. Being *patient-centred* has become a buzzword that administrators use to convince themselves and others that they are doing the right thing. The reality is that providing care that is truly *patient-centred* is very difficult. There is always room for improvement. However, a genuine, sustained commitment to providing *patient-centred care* is critical to excellent, program-based medical care.

At its core, *patient-centred care* involves looking at the medical experience through the eyes of the patient (and their loved ones). It is a very simple concept, but it is rarely invoked in the traditional Canadian medical system. Seeing the world through the patient's eyes allows for countless opportunities to improve the system—and by extension the experience that future patients will have.

Patient-centred care is not a passive process. It's an active process that includes strategies to acquire accurate feedback about what patients are actually experiencing. This feedback then needs to be acted upon. It is a continuous, iterative process. *Patient-centred care* is always a work in progress. However, programs that actively focus on patient care will almost invariably deliver a much higher level of care, often at a lower cost.

2. Teams must be formed around the episode of care (EOC).

Mrs. Johnson was an active 84-year-old woman who suffered a severe fracture dislocation of her ankle when she tripped going down the stairs in her home. She was taken to our emergency room, where the dislocation of her ankle was reduced and splinted. She was in a great deal of pain, and the nurse attending to her began giving her intravenous morphine, ordered by the emergency physician to help settle her pain. After an initial dose was given, the patient still rated her pain as a 7 out of 10, so a second does of morphine was administered. When she was transferred to the ward to await definitive surgery on her ankle, it was reported that she was "resting comfortably".

Eight hours later, she was found unresponsive and gurgling by one of the ward nurses. She was administered Narcan (a medication that counteracts the effect of morphine) and transferred to the Intensive Care Unit (ICU), where she was diagnosed with an aspiration pneumonia. The sedating effect of the morphine meant she was unable to reflexively protect her airway, and she had vomited some of her stomach contents into her lung. After three days in the ICU, her condition stabilized, at which point she underwent surgery to fix her fractured ankle. However, her hospitalization and overall recovery were markedly prolonged due to the effects of the aspiration pneumonia.

Despite the seriousness of this complication, the emergency physician who prescribed the morphine—and the nurse who administered it—never found out about the patient's ultimate results. From their perspective, it would naturally be important to ensure their patients' pain levels were well-controlled. If a similar patient presents to the emergency department again, they will likely render the same treatment.

This type of scenario is repeated over and over again within the Canadian healthcare systems. Operating room personnel violate sterile technique and do not see the resulting wound infection because it manifests itself weeks later. Physicians working in the hospital prescribe a medication to a patient and then discharge them—to be followed up by another physician—with no feedback on the effect of the prescribed medication. Disconnected from how care is delivered, administrators make personnel or protocol decisions that adversely affect care, yet they never see the direct effects of these decisions. A lack of consistent feedback is one of the many disadvantages of a department-based approach to care—as opposed to care that is organized around teams oriented to various EOCs (e.g., a fracture or trauma service line in this instance).

To optimize patient care, healthcare teams (doctors, nurses, physical therapists, administrators, etc.) of sufficient size and skill must be formed to coordinate care around either a set number of primary care lives or condition-specific EOCs. These teams (IPUs, programs, or service lines) must be organized in a manner that 1) facilitates easy communication among team members, 2) ensures a forum for sharing ideas and feedback, as well as reviewing results, and 3) incentivizes team members in such a way that they are all working towards a common goal.

These programs should ensure there is central oversight of the care that is provided—by a single individual who sees the EOC from start to finish and is held ultimately responsible for the results that are achieved. Furthermore, each team member should see their primary orientation and their job responsibility as being to their team—not their department. This type of team orientation is notably absent from the traditional, fragmented Canadian healthcare system.

Dr. Benson is a dedicated primary care physician who works in solo practice, aided by his assistant Jasmine. He works hard, seeing many patients each day. He regularly refers his patients out to be seen by physiotherapists, specialist physicians, and/or pharmacists. With few exceptions, he has never really met any of these individuals. He trusts they will do the right thing with his patients, but he has no way of knowing whether this happens. Furthermore, he would like to take more vacations, but when he does, he either has to temporarily shut down his practice or bring in a locum physician, who has no familiarity with his patients.

A team-based approach to patient management is also required in primary care. Delivering high-value primary care represents a unique and critical challenge to the healthcare system. The goal of addressing basic medical needs and providing coordination of care for more serious ailments—for a large roster of primary care patients—necessitates a multidisciplinary team approach; this will be outlined in more detail under principle #10.

3. Programs should focus on addressing clear goals, which need to be established by the health system.

When you get in your car, you need to know where you are going. You will often have many options as to the routes you may take to get to your destination. You may decide to take the fast route, the scenic route, or a route to try and avoid traffic. Or you may need to stop somewhere along the way. The route you choose will be affected by your goals in these areas. However, your decision-making is fundamentally predicated on having a clear destination.

Running a healthcare team is no different. It is essential to know where you are going: What are the specific goals for the team, program, or IPU? Furthermore, these goals—at least the big-picture goals—need to be generated by those governing the health system. They need to reflect the needs of the health system as a whole, rather than idiosyncratic goals developed by individuals or small teams in isolation.

This simple concept—having clearly-defined team goals that directly reflect the healthcare needs of the population—is absent in the management and organization of most healthcare systems in Canada. If overarching goals are present, they are often like those at my hospital—largely aspirational, formally stated but with no real meaning. Establishing teams, programs, or IPUs and directing them to pursue clearly-delineated goals would go a long way toward dramatically improving the healthcare system.

State clear goals, and stick to them. This simple idea has profound implications. It means saying *NO* to programs and individuals that are not aligned with the goals of the healthcare system's governing body.

4. Strong program leadership, which is responsible for the entire EOC, is essential.

An NHL team has clear leadership. The general manager is responsible for assembling a winning team and ensuring that it functions optimally. The coach is responsible for preparing the team for games and making decisions throughout that will hopefully lead to victory. Both the general manager and the coach actively oversee what is happening on the ice. Furthermore, they both realize they will ultimately be held responsible for the team's performance.

Healthcare teams also need clear leaders. These leaders must have specific responsibilities and powers. Specifically, team leaders must actually work *down on the playing field.* Leaders cannot be isolated from the actual care delivery process. They must have oversight of the entire EOC, and understand all of the aspects of care from start to finish.

Finally, they must be held accountable for the results of the EOC. Leaders of an EOC team cannot be mere figureheads. They must have the capacity to enact the needed change, and—like the coach and general manager of an NHL hockey team—they must be held responsible for the ultimate performance of the team.

5. A culture of excellence must be fostered among the entire team.

A minor miscue, such as a missed check, in the offensive end of the ice can start a chain reaction of events that can culminate in a goal for the other team. In hockey and in healthcare, little things make a big difference. A culture of excellence is essential.

21st century healthcare teams must be oriented towards excellence. This means doing the little things well *every* time. It means role-modeling performance standards, and working within a system where people on the team will be held accountable.

Excellence is achievable and is, in fact, fairly straightforward—when all members of the team are oriented to the same goals. This requires regular communication among team members, clear leadership, and an enjoyable, supportive culture. People—particularly people working in healthcare—usually want to do the right thing, but often they are placed in an environment where that is simply not possible.

6. Individual team members need to be held accountable for their performance.

What happens to an NHL player who plays poorly? Depending on his past history, he may be given some time to break out of his *slump*. He will often be given encouragement, and the coach may try and place him in a different position, where he can be successful and regain his confidence. If his poor performance persists, at some point he will be benched, demoted to the minors, or released. If his poor performance is due to a lack of effort or intensity, or he is behaving in a manner that undermines the team as a whole, the team's management will waste little time in ridding the team of this type of player. Every NHL player knows they will be held accountable for their individual performance.

Successful completion of an EOC requires teamwork. Often, the team is only as good as the weakest link. All of the following team members need to be held accountable for their performance: doctors who provide substandard care or effort, nurses who do not maintain appropriate standards, and administrators who do not provide an environment for the team to function well. This means remediation where possible, reassignment where viable, and dismissal if necessary. Without individual accountability for performance, the results of care from the team will be markedly affected.

In the traditional Canadian healthcare delivery model, coordinated teams are rarely formed. The organization of care is based on silos (nursing department, surgery department, medicine department, cleaning services, administration, etc.), which creates a fragmented delivery model. Without central oversight and with much closer alignment to his or her traditional silo, no one is really in charge. The resulting leaderless system for care means there is a distinct inability to hold any individual accountable for reasonable performance standards.

7. Outcomes must be independently measured.

The NHL measures numerous, objective statistics about every NHL team. They record which team won each game and how many points each team amassed during the season. Based on this, they determine which teams make the playoffs. Win four seven-game playoff series, and your team will be hoisting the Stanley Cup. While there are some subjective referee decisions, the NHL goes to great lengths to ensure rules are applied evenly, and the various outcomes for each team are measured objectively.

Similarly, outcome metrics for each player—such as goals, assists, penalty minutes, shots on net, and minutes played—are accurately recorded. Teams use this information, as well as other, more subjective data, to make player/personnel decisions—play them more, play them less, give them a new contract, send them to the minor leagues, or cut them from the team.

Governing healthcare bodies also need to collect accurate, objective outcome data on their various healthcare teams. In turn, these teams need to collect accurate data on their various team members. Just as there is a wide array of measurements that the NHL collects on its teams and players, there are many data points that can be collected about healthcare teams and their providers. Four broad categories of outcome metrics that are most important are 1) patient satisfaction, 2) patient outcomes, 3) adverse patient events, and 4) the cost of care delivery.

To be accurate, healthcare outcome metrics need to be measured independently. Outcome data that is collected by the healthcare team—without independent verification—will not be sufficiently accurate.

There are at least three reasons why recording accurate outcome metrics for healthcare teams is critical. First, these metrics are required to determine the relative success or failure of the team. Just as the number of points that a hockey team scores throughout a regular season can shed light on that team's performance (with respect to other teams), so too can healthcare teams be compared. Second, each team needs a robust continuous quality improvement (CQI) process; to do this requires hard, accurate outcome data. In the same way that a hockey team will make changes to address deficits they have identified, healthcare teams need to systematically improve their performance based on the outcomes they are achieving. Finally, outcome metrics can be used by team leaders to judge the relative performance of some of their providers—particularly physicians and those who are leading the team. Without accurate outcome measures, the care process and the associated team are working blindly.

8. Quality improvement initiatives should be incorporated into every program.

One of the hallmarks of any high-functioning team is continuous quality improvement. Time and time again, successful NHL teams and high-functioning businesses have demonstrated the critical importance of striving to always improve performance. This ethos must also be present within any successful healthcare team.

There are a variety of successful quality improvement tools that can be used to aid this process.[183] Tools such as a *lean thinking*, *Six Sigma*, and *total quality management* (TQM) can be used to create an iterative process that focuses on improving the team performance—by incorporating outcome data and involving members of the team itself. Any team that oversees a process that is characterized by numerous, often complex variables must have one or more formal quality improvement strategies. This is particularly true for healthcare, where adverse events can be catastrophic.

9. Healthcare providers should practice to the limits of their license.

Physicians are very expensive resources. High-value healthcare teams should not be paying physicians for services that can be rendered just as effectively by highly-trained—but less expensive—healthcare providers, such as nurse practitioners, registered nurses, physician assistants, and medical assistants.[184] When incorporated as part of a well-coordinated healthcare team, these types of allied healthcare providers can serve to dramatically decrease costs. And because they tend to work in a more standardized manner, they also often improve quality.

Healthcare screening, patient information intake, diagnosing and treating basic conditions, and facilitating patient education are all examples of essential healthcare services that often do not need to be performed by a high-priced physician. The ability to have healthcare providers "work within the limits of their license" is critical to the development of a cost-effective, high-quality healthcare system.

---

[183] Pinney SJ, Page AE, Jevsevar DS, Bozic KJ. Current concept review: quality and process improvement in orthopedics. *Orthopedic Research and Reviews*. 23 December 2015 Volume 2016:8 Pages 1—11

[184] The Future of Nursing: Leading change, advancing health. *Institute of Medicine*. DE Shalala (chair) 2011. http://iom.nationalacademies.org/Reports/2010/The-Future-of-Nursing-Leading-Change-Advancing-Health.aspx (Accessed January 2nd 2016)

10. Primary care delivery programs should be multidisciplinary, coordinated, and outcome-oriented.

Is it easier to coordinate primary care delivery for a group of 100 or a group of 20,000? The answer is that it is almost always easier to coordinate care for 20,000, and the reason for this has to do with variations in demographics.

Two groups of 100 patients are statistically likely to have wildly different levels of medical complexity. One group might be largely healthy one year, whereas the other group might (purely by chance) have three or four individuals suffering from life-threatening conditions, such as cancer—as well as 10 or more patients with serious chronic disease management issues, such as diabetes or heart failure. This can and does happen simply by random variation.

Two larger groups of 20,000 patients are likely to be very similar to each other in their demographics and their relative medical issues. Due to their large size, both groups are likely to have a similar percentage of very sick patients, as well as patients with specific chronic conditions. Furthermore, primary care organizations that manage large numbers of patients with specific conditions (e.g., cancer, shoulder problems, high blood pressure, heart failure, etc.) will find it cost-effective to develop specific programs to manage these patients. This will not be the case for smaller groups that have fewer patients with a specific condition. Larger primary care groups have the potential to create a variety of programs to address the common chronic conditions their patients will encounter—in a cost-effective and high-quality manner.

A multidisciplinary, team-based approach means that not every patient is going to be seen by a physician. In many instances, it will be just as effective for some patients to be managed by another member of the team, such as a nurse or physician assistant. He or she can deliver algorithmically-based care, while being overseen by the patients' designated primary care physicians. When done correctly, this renders care that is more personal, more effective, and less expensive.

Primary care teams need to divide up the labour associated with good medical care. Which individuals are best suited to perform which tasks? Perhaps it is that the group's licensed practical nurse is best positioned to coordinate the chronic disease management program for high blood pressure. All of these types of decisions can be made by the team leaders, with a view toward trying to determine how best to manage a large group of primary care patients.

Continuity of care is essential. Having a multidisciplinary, team-based approach to primary care delivery still means each patient will have their own primary care physician to coordinate their care. It also means each physician will be supported by other members of the healthcare team. This will allow him or her to ensure that each of their patients receives the required care. It also means that when a physician is away on vacation or at a conference, one of his or her colleagues can step in to help the other members of the team provide seamless care.

Each member of the team will be asked to "work to the level of their license," meaning physicians (and other members of the team) should not be doing work that can be done just as effectively by somebody who is a less expensive resource. If this team-based approach is employed in a coordinated, high-quality manner, many more patients can be taken care of, patient satisfaction will be improved, and overall cost will decrease.

11. Compensation should be aligned to promote high-value care.

NHL players, coaches, and managers are hired with the expectation that they will perform specific tasks. They are salaried, often with incentive bonuses that they will receive if they achieve certain landmarks.

This is not how compensation within the existing Canadian healthcare system works. Physicians are typically paid fee-for-service, receiving money for each fragmented aspect of care they provide. The more care they administer, regardless of whether it is actually needed or not, the more money they will make. Some physicians also receive stipends for various roles they may serve within the healthcare system. However, these are rarely tied to performance and often come to be expected. In contrast, nurses and other healthcare workers receive an hourly wage, regardless of the efficiency with which they work. Finally, most administrators receive flat salaries that are not dependent upon any performance metrics.

Reforming the Canadian healthcare system will require reforming the compensation system. If a healthcare team needs a surgeon to be in clinic two days a week seeing a set number of patients and to be in the operating room performing surgery on a certain number of patients another two days a week, the surgeon should be contracted in such a way that he or she must deliver these services. Patient satisfaction rates, low complication rates, and cost efficiency should be rewarded with productivity bonuses. Ideally, the entire healthcare team should receive productivity bonuses based on the overall performance of the team.

Research suggests that when employees work on commission, the compensation to adequately motivate them must be a minimum of 22% of their pay.[185] As such, it would seem prudent to have 30% or more of a physician's and/or administrator's compensation tied to the overall results of the healthcare team. Furthermore, there are ways to reward other members of the team for contributing to the achievement of overall team goals. Aligning the compensation system to promote team goals is one of the core principles in a modern healthcare system.

12. Programs that underperform should be reformed or eliminated.

Leading up to the 2010-2011 NHL hockey season, the Atlanta Thrashers were performing poorly, both on and off the ice—losing a reported 130 million dollars.[186] The owners, tired of losing money and recognizing that they could gain a financial windfall, announced the sale of the team on May 31, 2011 to the Winnipeg-based True North Sports and Entertainment (TNSE) ownership group. Subsequently, the new Winnipeg Jets were reborn.

Selling an NHL hockey team and moving it to another city has been relatively uncommon in the last 40 years; teams, in general, have been relatively stable. However, what makes up the team—the coach, general manager, president, and players—often changes dramatically. It is common for teams that finished at the bottom of the standings at the end of a season to be completely different within a few years. They

---

[185] http://theirf.org/research/incentives-motivation-and-workplace-performance-research-and-best-practices/147/

[186] http://en.wikipedia.org/wiki/Atlanta_Thrashers#cite_note-10

have a new general manager, a new coach, and new players; often, the only thing that has not changed is the team's uniform and the city they play in.

Governing bodies of healthcare must have the same capacity to invoke wide- scale change in poorly-performing teams—for two very important reasons. First, poorly-performing teams—rendering poor and/or expensive healthcare—are problematic, both for patients and taxpayers. Second, allowing poorly-performing programs to persist sends a clear message to others in the system: that poor care and lack of proper management are not only acceptable, but will be rewarded. This message is regularly sent in the present-day Canadian healthcare system.

From a management point of view, it will be easier for healthcare governing bodies to delineate goals—and parameters by which those goals need to be achieved—and then measure the results, while staying at arm's length from the actual teams. In this scenario, the easiest way to ensure that poorly-performing healthcare teams do not persist is to actually eliminate those teams. When whole programs are eliminated for underperformance, this sends a clear message to everyone else in the system as to the required performance standards. This is likely to only affect 5% or fewer of the teams, but is a critical concept. It clearly states to the healthcare system, as a whole, that high-quality and efficient performance is the standard that everyone must subscribe to.

Principles of Healthcare Teams: Summary

This section has outlined 12 principles, which should guide how Integrated Practice Units (healthcare teams) function within a modern medical system. It has argued how these teams should be organized: akin to how NHL hockey teams are organized. The unfortunate reality is that within most components of the Canadian healthcare system, this principle-based approach never gets past principle #2: *Teams must be formed around the EOC.*

Imagine if all of the goalies in the NHL were more closely aligned with each other than with their respective teams—and the same for the centers, forwards, defensemen, and coaches. This is akin to what typically happens in the Canadian healthcare system. Surgeons are aligned with surgeons, anesthesiologists are aligned with anesthesiologists, nurses are aligned with nurses, and administrators are aligned with administrators.

As seen through the eyes of patients, the EOC is not mirrored in the way that care delivery is actually rendered. All of these remaining principles are either moot or very difficult to implement—without reorganization to a team-based approach to care delivery. This change in system design must be initiated at the level of the governing healthcare body. It is impractical to think that doctors, nurses, and administrators will self-organize in this manner. It's simply not in their best interests to do so. However, with strong leadership from the governing body—leadership that is aligned with the principles that have been outlined for this group—healthcare teams can be assembled and high-quality care can be consistently delivered at a reasonable cost.

Principles for Doctors and Healthcare Providers

Doctors and other healthcare providers are the players that make healthcare work. With the changes inherent in 21st century healthcare delivery, providers need to understand that they now have different roles and responsibilities than in the past. Doctors need to be held accountable to new performance standards. The days of the lone physician toiling in isolation are becoming a thing of the past.

Like professional hockey, modern medicine is now a *team sport*. Teams need star players, but just like any team game, an individual player's actions must be subservient to the team and the team's goals.

The following principles should guide the actions and behaviors of modern physicians and healthcare providers.

1. Realize that times are changing.

The nature of healthcare delivery will change dramatically in the near future. The focus on value—and the associated reorganization of the system—will result in a medical landscape that looks very different than it has in the past. Change is scary, especially when it threatens to affect the careers and the lifestyles of those involved. However, for healthcare providers in general and physicians in particular, being a team player is no longer optional. Physicians in this new medical system are expected to not only join the team, but to help lead it. Those that embrace this concept will do well. Those that resist these changes are likely to find things increasingly difficult.

2. Be a good teammate. (Use healthcare providers to the limits of their licenses.)

As has previously been pointed out, physicians are expensive resources, and the healthcare system should not be paying for physicians when they can get the same, or better, service out of allied healthcare providers *working to the limits of their licenses*. However, these individuals need to work under the direct guidance of one (or more) physician(s). This means physicians need to be good teammates. They need to train, support, and provide feedback to those healthcare extenders who work with them as part of their team. They need to be role models. For many physicians, this responsibility will come easily; for others, it will take work.

3. Understand that "bad behavior" will be penalized, not rewarded.

It is essential that those running a health system not coddle bad physicians. Accepting, and in many instances rewarding, bad behavior sends the wrong message. It tells those working in the system that you can get ahead by acting in a manner that is contrary to the goals of the system as a whole.

What does it mean to be a bad physician? Traditional definitions— such as a lack of knowledge and skill, disruptive behaviors, and poor interpersonal skills—still apply. To these, a new category of *bad physicians* needs to be added: physicians that consistently act in a manner that is contrary to the goals of their healthcare team. The most talented surgeon or the smartest internal medicine physician may be a *bad physician*—if their actions undermine the quality and value that their healthcare team is delivering.

Anyone unwilling or unable to work as a productive part of the healthcare team should be considered a bad physician and treated accordingly. By this expanded definition, perhaps 10-20% of physicians would fall into this "bad physician" category. Fortunately, many can be remediated through retraining and a realignment of incentives. However, there are still likely to be at least 2-5% of physicians who will not be capable of remediation. These individuals should be excised from the healthcare system. Just as in professional hockey, what is best for the good of the team must trump the goals of individual players.

4. Physicians need to develop leadership skills.

Most NHL coaches and general managers are former players. Furthermore, they spend their time watching the game and interacting with the players on their team. They may not be on the ice when the game is played, but they know what the players are experiencing. Coaches and general managers are immersed in the actual game, not reading about it far away from the action.

Similarly, healthcare administrators must have at least one foot on the playing field. It is essential that those overseeing clinical programs and the various EOCs that they are facilitating understand all of the clinical elements required for them to be successful. They must also understand the various responsibilities of all of the players—and the potential ways in which breakdowns can occur. Like NHL coaches and general managers, only healthcare providers who are actively involved in providing care can have this intimate knowledge. Combined with accurate outcome metrics and basic management skills, this knowledge is required to lead a modern healthcare team.

From this definition, it is easy to understand that physicians are ideally positioned to assume these leadership roles in a modern healthcare system. However, to be effective in this new leadership role, they must acquire an additional skillset beyond those needed to practice clinical medicine at a high level. Healthcare organizations should seek out physicians and other healthcare providers with these skillsets and interests. Medical schools and residency training programs should understand that a physician's success may depend upon his or her ability to function as leaders of healthcare teams—and should prepare them accordingly. Management and leadership skills must be taught within their curriculum, both formally and through role-modeling.

5. Compensate physicians based on the value they add, not on historical norms.

Cataract surgery was once a complex endeavor that often required many hours. Due to the time and skill required to perform these procedures, compensation was set at more than $400 per procedure—when the provincial fee schedules were set in the early 1970s. Now, after many advances, uncomplicated cataract surgery takes 15 minutes or less, but the fee for the procedure has not been reduced accordingly. As a result of this and other vastly improved procedures, ophthalmologists are often the highest-paid medical specialty—with many specialists making well over $400,000 per year.[187]

One of the central reforms of the Canadian healthcare system has to be paying for outputs, not inputs. This is as opposed to continuing to do things because "that's how they've always been done." In addition to making no logical sense, this sentiment is also expensive and fosters fragmented, poor-quality medical care. Reforming physician compensation—by moving to contract or salaried positions with clear performance responsibilities—is mandatory in any movement to embrace the principles of modern healthcare organization.

6. Focus on the services required by physicians, not on the number of physicians.

It has been reported that there is a shortage of physicians in Canada. At the same time, 1 in 6 newly-trained physicians are unemployed or underemployed.[188] There may or may not be a shortage of physicians in Canada. However, trying to identify the number of actual physicians required to service the population is the wrong approach. A more effective approach would be to reframe the question: *What physician services are required?* There is a subtle but important difference between these two questions.

---

[187] How Much are Canadian Doctors Paid? Andre Picard. *The Globe and Mail* January 23rd 2013. http://www.theglobeandmail.com/life/health-and-fitness/health/how-much-are-canadian-doctors-paid/article7750697/ (Accessed January 2nd, 2015)

[188] http://news.nationalpost.com/2013/10/10/doctor-shortages-a-myth-nearly-one-in-six-new-medical-specialists-cant-find-work-report-suggests/

Consider two groups of orthopaedic surgeons, each working within a health system that needs them to provide orthopaedic care to its patients. One of the groups has five surgeons, and the other group has ten surgeons. Which group provides the most orthopaedic care?

At first glance, it might be natural to conclude that the larger group provides more services, but that may not be the case. Suppose that by choice, surgeons in the larger group are only in clinic one day per week and in the operating room another day per week—preferring to undertake other, perhaps more lucrative, activities during the remaining three workdays. Meanwhile, the five-man group is in clinic three days per week and in the operating room two days per week. In this scenario, the smaller group would be at least as productive as the larger group, in terms of patients seen and operations performed.

Similarly, wide variations can exist in the quality and cost of care. These types of scenarios are common within the Canadian healthcare system. This makes it difficult to understand what productivity you can expect from a specific number of physicians. The solution is simple: Focus on physician services and productivity, not on the actual number of physicians and other healthcare providers.

Patients: Roles and Responsibilities

"Patient-centred care" is a ubiquitous phrase within the Canadian healthcare system. Every hospital seems to claim they provide this type of care. The reality is that, in most instances, there is little that is truly "patient-centred" about the care that is delivered. Yet the concept of organizing care around the patient is valid. The Canadian healthcare system should primarily exist to service patients and their healthcare needs. Therefore, understanding the needs of our patients becomes essential.

In any new healthcare paradigm, the system must be responsive to the needs of patients and their families. However, patients themselves have a critical responsibility to act in a manner that allows the healthcare system to function well. There are certain principles that must guide each patient's behaviors. A healthcare system has a right to expect that patients will adhere to these principles for their own benefit—and for the benefit of the system as a whole.

1. Patients need to take responsibility for their health and their healthcare.

The vast majority of factors that determine whether an individual is healthy or not have nothing to do with their healthcare system. Living a healthy lifestyle—eating well, exercising regularly, refraining from smoking, and avoiding obesity—must be considered the responsibility of individuals, not of the healthcare system. Certainly, there are many things a healthcare system can and should do to facilitate appropriate behaviors in these realms, but individuals ultimately need to take responsibility for these areas—at least to the extent they are able to.

Individuals must also be proactive with respect to their healthcare. This means seeking out a primary care provider and working with this individual and his or her team to help foster preventive medical care, such as regular healthcare screenings (diabetes, colon cancer, etc.) and vaccinations. It also means actively collaborating with their primary care provider when a medical issue does arise.

2. Patients must be active participants in their healthcare.

Much of the healthcare system is predicated on patients and their families being active participants in treatment. Certainly there are scenarios, such as patients who have lost consciousness, where the system will take over. However, for most aspects of care, active participation by patients is essential if optimal outcomes are to be achieved.

Patients must actively seek out care. They need to ask questions. They need to think about how they would like to be treated, and what results they are looking for. This sort of proactivity helps those providing care understand the patient's goals. Having clarity when agreeing on the goals of care is usually the first step to getting the care that is needed. All too often, goals are not made clear, either because they are not stated by the patient or not asked for by the providers.

When this happens, healthcare is not patient-centred, and the subsequent results are often poor—in terms of patient satisfaction, quality of care, and cost. The system needs to ensure, as much as possible, that each patient's wishes are understood. However, patients play a critical role in this relationship, and must understand that active participation in their own care is essential.

3. Provide feedback on their experience.

Collecting accurate outcome measures is critical in 21st century medicine. The system will flounder without accurate feedback on the results of care. Patients need to be open to giving this kind of feedback. This requires honesty, including constructive criticism when asked. It also means proactively volunteering suggestions that could help the system as a whole meet the needs of future patients.

4. Recognize the limitations of the healthcare system.

Many patients have preconceived ideas about what ails them, and what they need to get better. Often these ideas are correct, but in some instances, they are misguided. Patients must understand that the healthcare system does not exist simply to meet any whim they happen to have related to their healthcare. Demands for inappropriate medications, unnecessary surgeries, and excessive time off from work are all regular examples of how patients' agendas are not in line with the goals of the healthcare system as a whole. Patients need to understand that these situations do occur, and when they do, the healthcare system is obliged to act in a way that supports the integrity of the system—not the specific whim of the patient.

Summary: Chapter 8

The NHL head office, all of the NHL teams, and each player make decisions based on well-known principles. The actual decisions may vary depending upon the circumstances. However, violating established hockey principles that underlie actions means courting disaster for the league, for teams, or for individual players.

The NHL—run by a strong, central, executive office—trumps the goals and wishes of any individual hockey team. The betterment of the league as a whole is more important than any single team. Similarly, a 21st century healthcare system— which is committed to delivering high-quality, cost-effective medical care to the patients it serves—must ensure that the goals and actions of the governing body trump the individual goals of teams—and particularly healthcare players, such as physicians.

Some of the core principles that the NHL relies on include having clear and specific goals, accurately measuring results, aligning incentives for the betterment of the league, promoting fairness and transparency, and ultimately having a high-quality, exciting brand of hockey. This chapter identifies 15 principles that those running the governing body of a healthcare system need to invoke to optimize the chance of the healthcare system being successful. One central principle for an integrated healthcare system is that there must be only one governing body coordinating the system—a group that truly represents the patients and the taxpayers.

A successful hockey team must focus on what it actually takes to win hockey games. It needs strong leadership, both on and off the ice; individuals who are held fully accountable for their performance; a culture of excellence; clear performance metrics; and a continuous striving for excellence and improved performance, based on the results they obtain.

Healthcare teams are equivalent to hockey teams in many ways. They need to have clear goals, based on patients' care needs. They need strong leadership that is not divorced from the healthcare playing field. Individual team members must be held accountable for their performance, and a culture of excellence must be fostered. 21st century healthcare delivery is now a team sport, and being consistently successful requires adherence to the 12 core principles outlined in this chapter to ensure team success.

Excellent teams require excellent players with a variety of skills. However, no individual player trumps the larger goals of the team itself. This has not always been the case in healthcare. This chapter emphasizes that healthcare teams need to take precedence over individuals, and it outlines the principles by which individuals working within a healthcare system should function.

Just as with the NHL, actions in healthcare should be guided by basic principles. These guiding principles do not lock the league, the teams, and the individual players into specific actions. But they must guide actions if success is to be achieved on the ice or in the healthcare arena.

Summary Points: Chapter 8

This chapter outlines a series of guiding principles that need to be invoked in order to deliver high-value 21st century healthcare. These principles are outlined as they pertain to three important elements:

1) a dominant *governing body* that organizes and is responsible for the entire system,
2) distinct types of *teams* oriented around primary care, service lines, or facilities, and
3) groups of *individuals* functioning within a health system (healthcare providers, administrators) to support the care of patients.

In the traditional Canadian healthcare system, the *governing body* is often less clearly delineated, as provincial health ministries may share (or abdicate) oversight of the system to regional health authorities or, in some instances, hospitals.

Principles that should guide the effective functioning of the governing body include:

1. Have a single governing body that actively manages the healthcare system from the patients' (and taxpayers') perspectives.
2. Have clear and specific patient and population outcome goals.
3. Promote patient-centred teams, NOT individuals.
4. Accurately (and independently) measure the results of care.
5. Pay for outputs, not inputs.
6. Align incentives.
7. Primary care should be the foundation of the healthcare system.
8. Ensure that care is coordinated across geography.
9. Embrace technology that improves efficiency and quality.
10. Respect physicians' (collective) autonomy, NOT physician's (individual) autonomy.

11. Eliminate "tollbooths" and "too big to fail."
12. Be open to change.
13. Minimize bureaucracy.
14. Promote transparency.
15. Keep politics out of healthcare.

To ensure that healthcare *teams* are facilitating the delivery of high-value patient care, the following principles should be invoked:

1. Actively strive for truly patient-centred care.
2. Teams must be formed around the episode of care.
3. Programs should focus on addressing clear goals, which need to be established by the health system.
4. Strong program leadership, which is responsible for the entire episode of care, is essential.
5. A culture of excellence must be fostered among the entire team.
6. Individual team members need to be held accountable for their performance.
7. Outcomes must be independently measured.
8. Quality-improvement initiatives should be incorporated into every program.
9. Healthcare providers should practice to the limits of their licenses.
10. Primary care delivery programs should be multidisciplinary, coordinated, and outcome-oriented.
11. Compensation should be aligned to promote high-value care.
12. Programs that underperform should be reformed or eliminated.

Doctors and other healthcare providers are the players that make healthcare work. With the changes inherent in 21st century healthcare delivery, physicians need to understand that they now have different roles and responsibilities than in the past.

The Canadian healthcare system exist primarily to service patients and their healthcare needs, but a healthcare system has a right to expect that patients will adhere to basic principles for their own benefit—and for the benefit of the system as a whole.

CHAPTER 9

Reforming the Canadian Healthcare System: Potential Solutions

September 2, 1972 was a day that changed Canadian hockey forever. On that day, at the hallowed Montreal Forum, the Soviet Union's national team defeated the Canadian team (comprised of NHL All-Stars) 7 to 3 in the first game of the Canada/USSR super series.

The best hockey players that Canada had to offer were totally outplayed. The Soviet team they encountered played like no team they had ever seen before. Their passing was impeccable, their fitness was outstanding, and their skill level was uniformly high. But most impressive was their teamwork.

This game was an impetus for disruptive innovation of Canadian hockey. The changes did not happen immediately. They occurred over a generation. However, the changes were dramatic. Professional hockey players began to train year-round, subtle skills were honed through hours of practice, and most importantly, the nature of what it meant to play team hockey was redefined.

Introduction: The Opacity of the Canadian Healthcare System

The Canadian healthcare system functions behind an opaque curtain. Therefore, it has not had this type of a public humiliation—an event that would force the system to be fundamentally reformed. Most citizens do not read studies such as the Commonwealth report, which suggests Canada has one of the poorest (and most expensive) healthcare systems in the developed world. Most people do not look at the federal and provincial budgets and see the amount of their tax dollars that is being spent on healthcare. Furthermore, the vast majority of the public does not have a meaningful encounter with the healthcare system in any given year; therefore, they do not have an opportunity to observe firsthand dysfunction within the system. The opacity of the Canadian healthcare system is unfortunate because the Canadian healthcare system needs an impetus for profound change.

This chapter explores what true healthcare reform might look like—and how it could be introduced. It is critical to emphasize that there are many potentially successful ways to reform a healthcare system. As outlined in Chapter 8, any change that adheres to the principles for running a 21st century healthcare system is likely be positive. What I present in this chapter is merely one potential version that could be successful. It is my hope that by outlining potential strategies for reform, it will provide a framework for real change—the type of change that will dramatically improve care and decrease cost.

There are two types of system changes: *evolutionary change* and *disruptive change*. Evolutionary change, as illustrated by the postal system analogy in Chapter 8, occurs when a system gradually and steadily improves in an incremental fashion. Disruptive change, as illustrated by the development of the internet represents a completely new paradigm. Canadians have and will continue to benefit from evolutionary change to their healthcare system. However, as has been outlined previously, the Canadian healthcare system is organized around a flawed design which acts as a roadblock. As such, a comprehensive solution will ultimately demand *disruptive* innovation. For Canadians to get the public healthcare system they deserve, the existing system will need to be fundamentally changed.

Evolutionary Change: Improving the existing Canadian healthcare system

The flawed design of the existing Canadian healthcare system creates a powerful argument for disruptive change—specifically building an entirely new second healthcare system from the ground up based on the principles of modern medicine. However, the practical realities are that, even in the best circumstances, a fundamentally new system for organizing and delivering healthcare could not be brought in rapidly or without significant growing pains.

Despite its many flaws, the existing system is not likely to disappear quickly. Therefore, active and aggressive steps need to be taken to incrementally improve the existing system. These improvements can and should be done while a new second public system—with the structural organization conducive to delivering good, modern healthcare—is built alongside the existing system.

The existing healthcare system could be improved more rapidly if four concepts were actively promoted within the system. First, look for ways to invoke the principles outlined in Chapters 6 and 8. Second, define specific, population-based healthcare goals, and promote programs—not individuals—to address these goals. Third, alter the funding model so the system is broken into smaller segments, none of which are "too big to fail." Finally, establish an independent, central means of collecting and utilizing accurate outcome metrics—metrics that can provide meaningful feedback that can then be used to modify care delivery to improve outcomes and decrease costs.

1. Where possible, invoke the principles of 21ˢᵗ century healthcare delivery.

The structure of the existing healthcare system prevents many principles of modern medicine from being invoked. However, there are some principles that can be applied, either partially or fully, to the existing system. Clear, specific, patient- and population-based outcome goals can be set and actively pursued. As much as possible, healthcare teams should be oriented around the EOC. Individuals should be held accountable for their performance within the system. Increased transparency can be promoted. A renewed focus on the outcomes of care and the various outcome metrics can also be promoted. These and other principles, which are outlined in Chapter 8, can help improve the existing healthcare system—when actually used.

2. Promote programs to address predictable, population-based healthcare needs.

The existing healthcare system is structured around inputs (doctors, nurses, administrators, equipment, medications, etc.). This input-oriented model makes it easy to forget the actual goals of the healthcare system. Taking a step back to identify predictable healthcare goals for a known population can help determine which services are actually required. How many patients in a specific population will need shoulder surgery in a given year? How many will suffer a heart attack? How many will be diagnosed with colon cancer? How many patients will need to be admitted to hospital for an acute medical condition or be placed on long-term medication for chronic illnesses?

When the healthcare population in question is large enough (e.g., provinces or health authorities), accurate answers can be determined for these population-based questions. When these questions are answered, it is not terribly difficult to take the next step and proactively determine which resources are required to provide these services. In most instances, the actual cost for providing these services in a coordinated manner is not prohibitively expensive, relative to what is already being spent. However, to provide the needed clinical care in these areas requires a coordinated programmatic approach—not a series of individual physicians each acting according to their own needs.

Any movement within the existing healthcare system to look at overall goals and address these goals programmatically is likely to improve the system. Focusing on programs forces those in said programs, and those overseeing these programs, to concentrate on what they are actually trying to achieve. This is contrasted with individual healthcare providers, who will invariably make decisions that are in their own best interests. Redirecting resources, such as operating time and clinic space, to programs and away from individual physicians is a practical and viable option, which would noticeably improve healthcare performance within the existing system.

3. Alter the funding model.

From bulk funding for healthcare institutions to private funding for prescription medication, the funding model requires bold transformation. First, the existing bulk-funding model—whereby hospitals and other institutions are given large yearly grants with relatively few measured performance responsibilities—should be changed. In the existing system, the primary means of cutting costs in the event of budgetary deficits largely involves across-the-board budget cuts.

If bulk funding is continued at all, a more effective means of allocating the resources would be to divide the system into subsections of organizations (programs or financial units), each budgeted between $10-50 million. Each of these financial units should have individual performance goals, and none should be *too big to fail*. Poorly-performing units from a financial or clinical point of view should be eliminated. This would not only save money; it would send a strong message to the remaining units: that performance outcomes are essential and that changes will be made to the healthcare system if needed.

An additional variation to this funding model would be to begin to move away from bulk funding altogether—and toward some form of activity-based funding of each program. This could be done by providing half of the funding to each program via a bulk grant, and then having the program bill the governing body (ex. Ministry of Health) for each EOC delivered to recoup the other half of the funding. This approach would allow funding to be partly based on productivity. It also leaves the option open of fostering outright competition between programs, which would greatly improve productivity and performance.

Consider two clinical programs that each provide care in the same area (e.g., shoulder surgery, colon surgery, acute inpatient hospitalizations, or outpatient mental health services). Imagine that each program treats the same number of patients (e.g., in the case of a shoulder surgery program, 4,000 new patient visits per year and 1,000 surgeries per year). Set the programs up so they are directly competing against each other. If more patients gravitate to one program, that program would get more funding. To keep costs fixed, set the amount of money that is available as the sum total of each half of the previously fixed budgets.

To do this effectively would of course require an accurate external assessment of patients entering the program, as well as the results of patients who did receive care. It would be unfair if one program were penalized for treating a disproportionate number of more complicated cases. Additionally, programs would need to be penalized financially for poor results or unnecessary treatments—a process that could be done via accurate external assessment of results.

Finally, if this type of movement away from bulk funding were instituted, it would need to be phased in gradually. For example, the ratio of bulk-program funding to activity-based funding would be 90%/10% the first year, 80%/ 20% the second year. Then an advance would be made by 10% each year until it was 50/50 in the fifth year.

Second, as examples from previous chapters have shown, medication funding requires a complete overhaul that is also based on performance and value. While a detailed discussion of potential prescription drug coverage strategies is beyond the scope of this chapter a comprehensive medication program is a necessary part of system reform. Given the importance of productivity and performance in ensuring the quality and value of the system, a medication program administered through a national organization and federally funded should cover only medications with a proven track record of effectiveness and cost efficiency, many of which will be low cost generic medications. Additionally, this type of national medication program could serve to help drive standardizations in care delivery by delineating appropriate indications to practitioners. This combined with objective metrics on prescribing patterns would help to standardize and improve care. Newer and more expensive medications that have not stood the test of time could still be prescribed by practitioners but would need to be paid for by patients or their private insurance as is presently the case today.

4. Establish an independent organization to collect accurate outcome metrics.

The existing Canadian healthcare system collects numerous metrics on almost all aspects of care. The Canadian Institute for Health Information (CIHI) was established to provide "essential information on Canada's health system."[189] They have an admirable mission and are making inroads into collecting useful data. Furthermore, almost every hospital collects local data.

However, many (if not most) of these collected metrics are of limited use. Often they are an inaccurate representation of what is actually happening, as in the example of altered length of care (ALC) patients and their bed utilization (covered in Chapter 2). Other metrics do not capture meaningful data (for example, implant costs that are not broken down by individual surgeons or associated programs). Yet accurate outcome metrics are critical for a highly-functional healthcare system. If those running a system do not know what the system is producing, how can they know what changes should be made to improve the system? Accurate outcome metrics in at least four domains are required. These domains include:

1. Patient satisfaction
2. Results of treatment (clinical outcomes)
3. Complication/adverse event rates
4. Costs of treatment

Presently, outcome metrics are often poor because they are collected by the same institutions that will be judged on these metrics. For example, many metrics are presently collated and analyzed by the CIHI, but the actual data collection is usually done locally—by the institution itself. Often it is not in the local institutions' best interests to have accurate metrics, or to have metrics that actually reflect relevant outcomes.

Most Canadian hospitals today have many individuals who are tasked with collecting various results of care. The reassignment of these individuals, or of their funding, to support an independent, central organization within each health system—which would accurately measure relevant outcome metrics and report these results to the governing body and the public—would be of tremendous benefit in improving the existing healthcare system.

---

[189] http://www.cihi.ca/CIHI-ext-portal/internet/EN/Theme/about+cihi/cihi010702

Disruptive Change: A strategy for creating an entirely new healthcare system

Changes such as those outlined above can serve to improve the existing healthcare system in an incremental manner. However, the organizational structure—on which the Canadian healthcare system is based—precludes many of the fundamental changes necessary to ensure that modern, team-based, cost-effective medical care is provided on a consistent basis. These are but a few of the major entrenched problems with the existing system that have previously been reviewed:

- Bulk funding of institutions irrespective of performance
- Fee-for-service compensation to physicians that rewards self-interested behaviors that are not team-oriented
- An administrative organization that ignores predictable, population-based healthcare needs
- A lack of accurate outcome metrics, which preclude meaningful feedback loops to enhance performance

Problems that stem from the underlying tenants of how the traditional healthcare system is organized include:

- Disconnected leadership by well-intentioned bureaucrats in the ministries of health
- Yearly bulk funding for care delivery via large hospitals, which creates no impetus to change
- Large payments to physicians on a non-competitive basis
- Lack of access to prescription drugs, and other non-insured services

As outlined in Chapter 5, these elements have a historical basis, which may have made sense at the time, but have become ensconced into the existing system. Practically, the foundation of this organizational structure cannot be changed in a meaningful way.

Many, if not most, individuals and groups within the Canadian healthcare system have carved out well-compensated niches, based on these entrenched ways of structuring healthcare delivery. These groups will fight change to this system as a means of self-preservation. Any impetus to introduce meaningful changes directed at the existing system will invariably be successfully rebuffed by those administrators, physicians, and healthcare workers who are presently running the system. They are not going to kill the goose that lays the golden eggs.

However, there is a way to create a new healthcare system—a system based on recognized principles of delivering modern medical care. The solution: *build a second, parallel public system and watch it supplant the existing system over time.*

If you would like to change an entrenched, complicated organizational structure, a direct frontal assault is usually not the best approach. People, especially people in large groups, naturally resist change, as well as the unknowns that change brings. This is especially the case when large, powerful organizations see change as diminishing or eliminating their power—along with the associated, lucrative career opportunities that this power brings. This would certainly be the case with any meaningful change to the structure of the Canadian healthcare system.

The issue is somewhat akin to curriculum reform at a medical school. What are the strategies for completely changing the way a medical school teaches its students? It turns out that deciding how students should be taught in order to increase the effectiveness of their education is substantially easier than determining how to introduce an entirely new curriculum to an existing, organizational structure. By forcing a major upheaval onto a skeptical and resistant faculty, many curriculum reforms have been unduly painful; some have even failed.

A much less painful and ultimately more effective approach is to build a second, parallel curriculum and have a small number of students (e.g., 5%) go through this curriculum in the first year. Each year, as students and faculty see the merits of the new curriculum, more students are added to the new pathway. Once 30-40% of the students are involved in a new curriculum, it is easy to flip the systems and eliminate the original curriculum. This is the approach Harvard Medical School took in 1985 when it fundamentally changed the paradigm of their curriculum—a new approach to medical education for the first time in more than a half-century.[190] An analogous *second pathway* approach offers the key to truly reforming the Canadian healthcare system.

---

[190]   http://www2.ed.gov/about/offices/list/ope/fipse/lessons2/harv-med.html

Building from the Foundation Up: A proposal for a new healthcare system based on the principles of modern medical care delivery

What might a new, high-quality, efficient, cost-effective, modern healthcare system look like? There are many potential solutions to this question. Adherences to the four core pillars of a modern healthcare system, as well as the other principles of 21st century healthcare delivery, are necessary for any model to be successful. Such a system must have clear goals based on population needs; it must practice *population-based healthcare*. Care must be delivered in a coordinated, team-based manner. Individuals must be held accountable for their performances. Accurate outcome metrics must be used to provide feedback on the system, so that accountability and continuous improvement is a defining feature of the new system. Finally, the system should fund *outputs*: the final results of care, not merely inputs to the system.

Incorporation of all the principles outlined in Chapter 8 is necessary to ensure that a new system consistently delivers high-quality care at a reasonable cost. What follows is a proposal for a public healthcare system that could run parallel with the existing system—supplanting it over time, as the quality and performance of this new system attracts more and more patients and government funding.

The proposed healthcare system would actually be a series of systems—at least one system per province, and perhaps more if health regions were designated as *governing bodies*.[191] This new system would be principle-based. Primary care would be at the core of this new system, and care would be delivered through team-oriented medical homes. Major medical issues, such as those requiring in-hospital treatment or surgeries, would be provided via *service lines* (programs) oriented around specific EOCs—not via individual practitioners oriented toward fragmented departments. Finally, hospitals and other sites where care is delivered would compete for patients, thereby demanding that these institutions—as well as patient-centred medical homes (primary care)

---

[191] Unless the federal government introduced a new single nationwide healthcare system, each new "system" would be introduced by respective provincial governments. References to "new system" and "second pathway" therefore refer to a parallel healthcare systems that *each* provincial government would initiate.

and service lines (specific programs)—compete with each other to ensure value is optimized.

Additional principles would be invoked throughout this new second pathway. Tollbooths—individuals who play an isolated but critical role in care delivery—would be eliminated. Instead, these critical service providers would be incorporated as key members of the larger service line. Outcome metrics would be gathered to assess the results of care, complication rates, patient satisfaction, and costs. These metrics would be collected by an independent group to ensure accuracy. Publicly reported outcome metrics would serve to shine a bright light on the results the system achieved, both good and bad—thus serving as a foundation for continuous improvement of quality.

No individual or group within this new system would be too big to fail. By dividing the system into small sub-segments, each with clear goals, it will not be possible for individuals or groups to shirk their responsibility for providing high-quality, cost-effective care. Competition among primary care practices, service lines, and hospitals will be essential within this second pathway.

Finally, this new second pathway requires new management. Running a healthcare system requires leaders who can and will make difficult decisions. They need to be given both the formal and cultural authority to make these types of decisions. These healthcare leaders should be rewarded or penalized appropriately, based on their performances. As such, the system cannot be directly run by government employees, although the government must ultimately be responsible for the system's performance.

Four Core Elements

This new system would be organized around four core elements. A single governing body would run the system, and the actual care would be delivered via an interplay between the three other elements: patient-centred medical homes (PCMH), service lines for specialty care, and hospitals and other facilities for care delivery.

1. *Governing body.* This powerful, mission-focused single entity would be responsible for the system's performance and day-to-day management.
2. *Patient-centred medical homes (PCMH)* –also known as *primary care medical homes.* A collection of "medical homes" would deliver most (90+ percent) medical care to those in the system, via a coordinated, team-based approach.
3. *Service lines for specialty care.* Service lines or programs organized to provide coordinated EOCs for specific conditions would provide medical care for those more complicated conditions and situations that cannot be easily handled by the PCMHs.
4. *Hospitals and other facilities for care delivery.* The most complex care will require hospitals and other facilities. These centers will compete for patients, based on service and cost.

The remainder of this chapter will expand on these core elements.

The Governing Body: Leadership in the New System

The NHL head office runs the league. Their overarching goal is to improve the overall product of the league in its entirety. The more successful the NHL is in attracting fans to watch the games, the more revenue and other forms of success the league as a whole and all the teams achieve. Strong mission-driven leadership of the league as a whole is critical. Running a healthcare system is no different.

The roles and leadership characteristics of those who will successfully govern this new system will need to be dramatically different than those who are presently governing the existing healthcare system. They will need to function at arm's length from the political process. Leaders will regularly need to make and enforce hard decisions; as such, they should be appropriately compensated when they are successful and fired when they are not.

Performance accountability at all levels will be paramount in this new system. There will need to be a small, highly-functional executive overseeing the new system, with an absence of middle management. Each individual functioning in a leadership capacity must have some direct connection with the healthcare playing field. This new system will need to be run like a business, arguably the most important business our society has—taking care of the health of our fellow citizens.

What follows is one potential strategy for implementing a new public healthcare system in Canada—a system built from the ground up and based on the principles of delivering good, modern medical care. If such a system is nurtured and given the opportunity to succeed, in time it will supplant the traditional Canadian healthcare system. Implementation of this system would be an example of disruptive innovation. It would fundamentally change the way healthcare is organized, administered, and funded.

Undoubtedly, there are other ways that fundamental healthcare reform could be introduced. However, I hope that discussion of this possible solution will stimulate a conversation that will lead to meaningful system change. What follows is a review of the core ideas that would underlie the governing body of this new, second public system.

1. Form a Crown corporation (or equivalent) to run the new healthcare system.

Politics and healthcare do not mix. Building a new hospital in a politically important community or placating the needs of a vocal and well-organized minority of citizens may be a politically astute maneuver, but in many instances, these actions undermine the healthcare system as a whole. Yet these types of politically motivated decisions happen all the time within the government-run Canadian healthcare system.

An arm's-length corporation is needed to ensure that decisions are consistently made in the best interest of the system, not of specific individual players. This corporation needs to be focused on longer-term goals, not the next election cycle. Certainly, on a regular basis, they must be responsible to the citizens via the government. However, the day-to-day and month-to-month decision-making needs to be at arm's-length from the political process.

In Canada, there is precedence for the formation of a Crown corporation to run an organization that provides an essential public service. Both the Canadian Broadcasting Corporation (CBC) and the Bank of Canada run via government funding and with a government mandate—but with considerable independence from the government.[192,193] Without an organization that has independent leadership and autonomy, the ability to be successful will be limited. This is a major issue within the existing healthcare system. Healthcare leaders need to be able to make the hard decisions that best serve the long-term interests of the healthcare system.

2. Ensure leadership excellence.

Leaders of this new system—those on the executive level—must be highly skilled in business strategy, negotiations techniques, and medical care delivery. They will face strong challenges from large, powerful, self-interested organizations, such as doctors, nurses, and administrators. They must be prepared to meet these challenges, using high-level executive skills. Their focus must be on the end goals of high-quality, cost-effective healthcare for those that are treated within their system.

As previously stated, healthcare leaders, especially those at the executive level, must be held accountable for their performance. As such, those who are successful must be well compensated—with executive compensation set at a level equivalent to, or above, those of the highest paid physicians. Leaders that are not successful or consistently underperform must be relieved of their duties. Those leading the system must be transformative, not mediocre. The financial cost of paying for excellence at the executive level will pale in comparison to the money that they will save the system overall.

---

[192] https://en.wikipedia.org/wiki/Canadian_Broadcasting_Corporation (Accessed January 3rd 2016)

[193] http://www.bankofcanada.ca/about/#who-runs-the-bank (Accessed January 3rd 2016)

3. Organize care delivery around programs that compete.

Competition between health system programs will be essential. The proposed healthcare system will be centred around programs to provide optimal primary care to the population, as well as programs to deliver high-quality specialty care through established service lines. The logistics of these elements will be outlined in the next sections.

Numerous *patient-centred medical homes* will be established and funded to deliver primary care to groups of between 10,000 and 30,000 patients. Each medical home will be funded separately. Those medical homes that underperform, either because they incur excessive costs or because they fall short on quality metrics, should be given a small window of time to remediate. Those that fail to improve to an acceptable standard should be dropped.

Similarly, service lines to address more advanced clinical problems (e.g., musculoskeletal care, endocrine issues, and abdominal problems) will be funded independently and assessed based on their outcome metrics. Those medical homes and service lines that perform well will get more patients and more funding; those that do not will have to close or undergo reorganization. Internal competition to optimize value will be one of the defining features of this new healthcare system. Accountability based on accurate outcome metrics for PCMHs, service lines/programs, and facilities will be to the governing body. Clear goals will need to be set for each IPU entity, as well as a clear reporting structure within the governing body, and transparent objective evaluations on a regular basis. Just as a professional hockey team knows their place in the standings and the various metrics surrounding their performance so too should healthcare teams (IPUs).

Patient-Centre Medical Homes: Providing comprehensive, primary care to the population

Every professional hockey team has clear goals. To achieve these goals, they know they will need talented players. However, more critically, their individual players must play together as a team—functioning as a highly-integrated unit. The goals of the team itself must supersede those of the individual players. Players understand this reality. They also understand they will be held accountable for their performance. Furthermore, teams use accurate outcome data to assess their performance. This includes basic metrics such as wins, losses, point totals and their place in the overall standings. Additionally, it includes more granular metrics that the team's management use to accurately assess the performance of the team and the individual players.

Whether it be a primary care program (providing basic, primary care delivery to a large group of patients) or a specialty care service line (tasked with delivering the most complex types of care), a healthcare team needs to function using the same paradigm as a professional hockey team. Clear, population-based, group healthcare goals defined by the governing body are essential. Individual excellence among the providers is necessary, but not sufficient. The goals of each healthcare team must trump those of the individual players (doctors, nurses, and administrators). Outcome metrics, both basic and detailed, must be accurately recorded and used to improve the process and determine personnel decisions.

The next two sections outline what a new healthcare system would look like for healthcare teams—those delivering primary care services, and those establishing service lines (programs) to provide more complex patient care.

Team-based primary care delivery as the bedrock of the system

How does a healthcare system ensure that primary medical needs are met for a large population (20,000 or more patients)? It turns out the answer is surprisingly straightforward. However, to actualize this remedy requires a fundamental paradigm shift in how medical care is delivered. Primary care delivery via coordinated *medical homes* represents a potential solution. A solution that is gaining traction in modern healthcare systems, including in Canada.[194]

---

[194]   Gutkin C. Adapting the medical home concept to Canada. *Canadian Family Physician*. March 2010 vol. 56(3) 300. (Accessed January 3rd 2016)

First and foremost, any new medical system must place the delivery of primary medical care at its heart. A good primary care medical program will be able to treat 90+% of patient problems in the medical system at any given time. Furthermore, when done well, it ensures that high-quality medical care is delivered in a coordinated and cost-effective manner, both with respect to primary care and more complicated care – in both urban and rural communities.

The Canadian medical system, with its single-payer and central oversight, is ideally set up to have primary care serve as the foundation of the medical system. However, for many years, primary care practitioners have been treated as second-class citizens within the healthcare world. The fee-for-service compensation system that has dominated primary care reimbursement encourages—some would argue demands— short, superficial patient visits. Rushed patient visits do not allow for meaningful healthcare coordination. Any new healthcare system based on modern principles must emphasize primary care—usually via the establishment of coordinated medical homes for primary care delivery, in order to facilitate an effective way to achieve the system's primary care goals.

So what is good primary care? And by extension, what resources are required to provide this care? Primary care is the treatment of all basic and common medical conditions, as well as the provision of preventive medicine and the coordinated management of many chronic diseases. It ensures that all citizens have healthcare providers, who can diagnose and treat basic medical conditions—and who can then help coordinate their treatment if more complicated conditions arise. Good primary care management oversees clinical pathways and programs to ensure that patients are receiving excellent care.

This means patients receive the correct medications, have their chronic conditions (such as diabetes and high blood pressure) looked after in a systematic manner, and receive common specialty care (e.g., dermatologic, musculoskeletal, psychiatric, and geriatric problems) in a timely manner—often by specially-trained healthcare providers under the oversight of the primary care program. Effective, coordinated primary care programs will also ensure that common acute conditions (e.g., flus, urinary tract infections, and ankle sprains) are managed by providing extended office hours, eliminating the need for walk-in clinics and the expensive, fragmented care they provide.

So what are *patient-centred medical homes* (PCMH), and how do they deliver this type of care at a reasonable, per capita cost? A PCMH is a form of physician-led, team-based healthcare. Its goal is to provide coordinated, cost-effective primary medical care to a large number of patients. This is accomplished by:

1. *Treating large numbers of patients*
2. *Working as a coordinated healthcare team*
3. *Developing programs for common conditions*
4. *Instituting innovative quality and process improvement initiatives*
5. *Employing a fundamentally different compensation model*
6. *Accurately assessing the outcomes of care*
7. *Promoting patient responsibility within the medical home*
8. *Ensuring clear leadership, which is held accountable*

Each of the above eight concepts will now be reviewed in more detail to give a clearer picture of what an effective PCMH looks like.

1. Treating large numbers of patients

The effectiveness of a PCMH is predicated on treating large numbers of patients. PCMHs must manage large numbers of patients (10,000, or ideally more than 20,000 patients) to be successful. The reason for this is that large numbers of patients create predictability and allow for economies of scale. The medical issues of a large group of patients are predictable year after year.

This is not the case for a single physician working in an isolated practice, managing 1,000 or even 2,000 patients per year. In this situation, there would be too much annual variation. However, as the number of patients increases to 10,000 or more, this variation decreases considerably. This is the premise behind population-based medical care. It is possible to predict, with a high degree of accuracy, the types of patient issues that need to be treated.

As an example, consider a chronic disease management program. In a typical primary care population of 20,000 people, 6.8% (1,360 patients) will have diabetes, and 38.9% (529 patients) of these patients will have poorly controlled diabetes.[195,196] In traditional primary care practices, patients with uncontrolled diabetes are often lost in the system—showing up later with end-stage conditions, such as renal failure, loss of sight, or foot infections that require amputation. Those who are not lost in the system are often referred out for specialized care via an endocrinologist. With an in-house PCMH diabetic program, these patients will be proactively followed, and when they do need specialized care, they will initially be referred to an in-house physician with diabetes expertise.

Large numbers of patients allow for the benefits of economies of scale. By knowing with accuracy what conditions need to be treated, high-quality, cost-effective programs can be developed for patients. Diabetes, high blood pressure, shoulder problems, and a host of other clinical conditions can be managed by specific programs housed within the PCMH. The ability to create coordinated programs within a PCMH is one of a host of administrative, financial, and practical advantages to treating a large number of patients in a coordinated manner.

2. Working as a coordinated healthcare team

Patients within a PCMH are assigned their own primary care physician—a physician who manages their medical conditions and helps them navigate the healthcare system when they have more complex medical problems. However, this physician does not work in isolation. He or she would work closely with one or more healthcare extenders, such as a physician assistant (PA) or a nurse practitioner (NP). Together, the physician and his or her team would see at least twice as many patients as the physician could working in isolation.

Evidence-based algorithms and physician oversight ensure that patients get optimal care from the physician extenders on the team. Furthermore, as most PCMHs will have 6 to 10 physicians working

---

[195] http://healthydebate.ca/2013/05/topic/managing-chronic-diseases/canadian-diabetes-strategies-under-fire-as-diabetes-rates-continue-to-rise

[196] http://www.ncbi.nlm.nih.gov/pubmed/25451895

within the medical home, there will always be a partner physician available to assist patients, should their designated primary care physician be away or unavailable.

The team-based concept of a PCMH also offers a potential solution to ensuring rural and underserved populations have adequate access to primary care. With the increased use of telemedicine, the large group of patients that are managed by a single PCMH would *not* need to all be within one geographic community. Using telemedicine and an in-person community outreach program, PCMHs could be developed to provide primary care for patients in groups of smaller communities—including rural communities where physician recruitment and retention has often been problematic.

These concepts can also be applied to seniors' care, and those in long-term care (LTC) and assisted living facilities who could be managed effectively by the team-based approach of a PCMH. Seniors could be monitored and proactively treated using telephone or telemedicine resources by health providers working as part of the PCMH team. Similarly, by bringing LTC patients under the umbrella of a PCMH team and applying innovative and effective care strategies (ex. virtual monitoring, telemedicine, standardized care paths, etc) care can be improved and costs decreased in this tenuous and resources intensive patient population. Furthermore, situating seniors and LTC patients within a PCMH would facilitate more proactive longitudinal care for these patients and allow for proactive identification of bed and other healthcare resource requirements.

To facilitate team-oriented care, each PCMH would have a single, integrated electronic medical record (EMR) that will allow everyone in the medical home to understand each patient's medical issues and present treatment goals. In addition to physicians and healthcare extenders, other individuals that may make up the PCMH include administrators, pharmacists, physical therapists, healthcare navigators, and tech-support personnel. Those leading the PCMH would have wide leeway to hire any individual that could effectively serve the mission of the medical home. The PCMH, led by the partner physicians, would delineate the services their patients need and, using a team-based approach, would determine the best ways to meet the predictable needs of their patient population.

3. Developing programs for common conditions

One of the true strengths of a primary care medical home is that innovative programs can be developed to reduce cost and/or improve the quality of services provided. Costs can be reduced by having less expensive healthcare providers (nurses, physician assistants, medical office assistants, etc.) oversee routine but important healthcare activities—such as insuring up-to-date vaccinations; monitoring chronic conditions like high blood pressure or diabetes; or coordinating screening for at-risk patients.

Formal programs can also be developed within the medical home, made possible by the large size of the organization. Potential programs could include:

- Chronic disease management programs (e.g., high blood pressure, congestive heart failure, and diabetes)
- Specialty clinic programs (e.g., musculoskeletal problems, sinus problems, and dermatology problems)
- A navigator program for those who are facing complicated and serious medical conditions, such as a cancer diagnosis
- A complex patient management program
- In-house physiotherapy
- An in-house pharmacist employed to facilitate specific patient needs
- A fully integrated patient portal to allow email access between patients and healthcare providers
- A telemedicine program to allow certain types of appointments to occur online
- Outreach programs that would use telemedicine and visiting providers to extend primary care to rural and underserved areas

As an example, a specialty musculoskeletal screening program could be introduced to a PCMH, led by one of the healthcare providers with an interest and expertise in musculoskeletal conditions. Rather than wait many months to see an orthopaedic specialist, this type of program would allow patients quick access to an initial assessment by a musculoskeletal expert. Similar programs for abdominal issues, dermatological issues, head and neck issues, or any of a number of common specialty issues could be developed.

While these types of programs could be run under the leadership of one of the medical home's physicians, bringing in a specialist—to consult, on an expedited basis, with a subsection of the home's patients—would be a relatively easy extension of this type of program. By fully understanding the primary care needs of the patient population of each PCMH, those leading the organization can use their knowledge and creativity to develop unique and cost-effective programs—to ensure patients receive the care they need.

4. Instituting innovative quality and process improvement initiatives

Instituting programs to facilitate improved access to specialty care within the PCMH is just one example of the type of process-improvement program that could be implemented. A continuous review of the PCMH, including what is working and what needs improvement, would be a critical part of this type of team-based care. Each PCMH would be expected to form a quality improvement team that would meet regularly. This team would be made up of representative members (physicians, NPs, PAs, administrators, etc.) of the PCMH.

There are a variety of quality improvement (QI) initiatives they could promote (such as lean thinking, Six Sigma, total quality management, and root cause analysis covered in Chapter 6), depending upon the specific need that was identified. One such initiative that is representative of this type of QI approach is *Patient and Family Centered Care Methodology (PFCC)*. PFCC is a six-step, team-based approach to QI, which is centered on seeing the care delivery improvement from the point of view of the patient and their family, and on instituting changes that improve the process.[197]

There are many improvements PCMHs can make to the delivery system, which will achieve the *triple aim* of improving care, decreasing

---

[197] DiGioia AM, Greenhouse PK: Care experience-based methodologies: performance improvement roadmap to value-driven health care. *Clin Orthop Relat Res.* 2012;470(4):1038-1045.

costs, and improving the health of the population they oversee. Group education classes could be created to help facilitate patient education on common conditions. Coordinated group physiotherapy sessions for frequent musculoskeletal complaints (low back sprains, rotator cuff tendonitis of the shoulder, and/or osteoarthritis of the knee) can offer rapid access to therapy with no or minimal out-of-pocket cost. A telemedicine program, using readily available internet resources, can allow many patients—who would otherwise need to take a half day of work off for a doctor's visit—to be treated remotely. Interactive computer programs, using computer adaptive technology, can be employed to perform an initial screening assessment on patients—to ensure all diagnoses are obtained and that there is improved standardization of care. Shared decision-making tools can be used when patients are confronted with difficult treatment decisions, so that each patient is adequately informed and can therefore make the best decision.

These are just a few of the many potential processes and quality initiatives that could be instituted. Essentially, anything that improves the primary care delivery in a cost-effective manner can be quickly introduced.

5. Employing a fundamentally different compensation model

The implementation of this type of PCMH requires a fundamentally different funding model and a different means of compensating physicians. To facilitate this change, the governing body of the healthcare system would essentially purchase primary care from a PCMH. For example, they might purchase the management of 20,000 primary care lives for a 12-month period. This would not be a bulk payment that is irrespective of performance. There would be clear performance metrics tied to this payment, including minimum patient satisfaction and quality-of-care standards.

Furthermore, PCMH could generate more income if they could demonstrate that their per capita costs were lower than average. This would encourage the development of programs to effectively manage chronic diseases, so that expensive hospitalizations and surgeries could be minimized. Similarly, expert care in specialty areas that could be provided less expensively (and more quickly) via the PCMH would be rewarded.

Physicians working in a PCMH would be paid differently. They would be employed by the PCMH. The standard fee-for-service compensation model for primary care physicians simply does not work. It rewards poor, high-volume care and penalizes high-quality, patient-centred care. Rather, physicians would be paid a baseline salary by the PCMH. This salary would be determined by the number and complexity of patients that they were overseeing. In addition, they would be given the opportunity to receive regular bonus payments (ex. quarterly) if they, and the PCMH, met objective productivity, quality, and patient satisfaction standards.

Depending on a specific physician's practice, it would be expected that they would coordinate the care of between 1,500 and 3,000 patients. Patients would be risk-stratified; physicians overseeing a disproportionate number of elderly patients with multiple medical problems would not be at a disadvantage, compared to those physicians treating mostly younger, healthy patients.

Furthermore, bonuses of up to 35% of their total compensation would be available. These would be based on productivity, patient outcomes, and cost-effectiveness. This incentive structure would be organized in such a way that it would not be the norm for a physician to receive all of the bonus compensation for which he or she is eligible. Rather, it would be expected that bonuses representing approximately 50% of the eligible incentive payments would be the norm. In many instances, it would be expected that involved physicians might not qualify for a bonus in any given quarter. However, it would be very transparent as to who was eligible and how somebody achieved a bonus. The incentive structure would be designed to encourage high-quality, efficient care and to reward innovations that improve the PCMH.

6. Accurately assessing the outcome of care

Accurate outcome metrics will be key to the long-term success of any PCMH. A robust electronic medical record will provide regular diagnostic and treatment metrics that will allow the leaders of the medical home to make appropriate management decisions. What are the most common diagnoses that are being made? What are the most common treatments that are being utilized? Is there a seasonal variation to these diagnoses? Monthly or even weekly metrics that are automatically culled from the electronic medical record will help guide management decisions.

Accurate, independently-acquired outcome metrics will be additionally critical to the success of any medical home. These metrics will cover:

- Patient satisfaction
- Results of clinical treatment
- Complication / adverse event rates
- Cost of care
- Volume of care provided

Together, these metrics will provide critical feedback for the leaders of the medical home to improve its care and performance. They will help determine productivity bonuses, as well as possible punitive actions for the PCMH. This would include eliminating the funding, and thereby shutting down, PCMHs that are significantly underperforming, compared to competing medical homes.

7. Promoting patient responsibility within the medical home

Being a patient affiliated with a medical home will offer improved healthcare delivery to those individuals. With these advantages comes certain patient responsibility. Patients will be expected to be active and proactive participants in their healthcare—as much as they are able to. They will be expected to work with their treating physicians in a co-operative manner.

Furthermore, they will be expected to obtain all their medical care through the PCMH. For example, if they seek medical care outside of the medical home, such as through a walk-in clinic, they will risk being expelled from the PCMH. This is because the PCMH will be ultimately responsible for the overall healthcare costs associated with each patient. The corollary is that if patients are unsatisfied with the performance they are receiving within the specific PCMH, they can easily leave. An exodus of patients from one PCMH to another will invariably spell doom for the less popular PCMH.

8. Ensuring clear leadership, which is held accountable

Each PCMH will have a responsible *ownership* party, which is held ultimately accountable for the clinical and financial performance of the PCMH. It would be expected that, in most instances, PCMH ownership would come from an individual physician or a group of physicians, who decide to form their own PCMH. However, a business entity or an existing healthcare organization, such as a hospital, may also choose to establish a PCMH.

In each of these scenarios, it would be expected that the day-to-day decision-making of a PCMH would be led by a physician or council of healthcare providers who are actually practicing medicine. PCMH teams will remain relatively small, so bureaucracy will be minimized. If something needs to be done to improve care, those leading the PCMH must make this happen with a minimum of bureaucracy.

PCMH ownership groups—whether they be physicians, healthcare organizations, or businesses—would be given wide latitude as to how they organize the PCMH. This would include who they employ and how these individuals will function, provided they adhere to all applicable rules (provincial and federal, healthcare and employment).

Innovative solutions to administrative and clinical problems that improve outcomes and decreases costs will be rewarded. Inefficiency and waste will be penalized. It would be expected that between 5-10% of medical homes would fail. Ultimately, each PCMH ownership group would bear the full responsibility for the success or failure of each individual PCMH.

Service Lines for Specialty Care: An EOC-based approach for more complex care

How would a new *second pathway* healthcare system, based on disruptive innovation of care delivery, provide healthcare to Canadians for the most involved and serious of conditions (the 5-10% of medical problems that cannot be managed by primary care teams)? The logical solution is to build a team around the patient's EOC; this is also known as a *service line* or *programmatic* approach. To someone outside the healthcare system, the solution is not exactly new, and it may not seem particularly innovative. However, the movement toward a coordinated, team-based approach to the EOC would represent a radical departure from the traditional, fragmented approach to delivering specialty and complex patient care, which is still ubiquitous within the Canadian system.

One of the early examples of this model of care is a distinctly Canadian institution—the aforementioned Shouldice clinic. By focusing on one clinical condition (hernias) and by organizing care so that everyone working there is oriented toward the same goal, they have consistently achieved outstanding results that have given them a well-deserved, worldwide reputation for excellence. Having an entire team with a single clinical focus is an intuitive organizational approach. Everyone works toward clearly-identified, common, patient-centric goals. This is combined with a high volume of care, so that true clinical expertise is developed throughout the experience.

Reorienting care delivery around service lines to address specific clinical conditions (e.g., colon cancer, shoulder problems, sinus problems, and kidney problems) solves most of the problems inherent in traditional care delivery models. The service line-based approach is now common at other major institutions. Both the Cleveland Clinic and the Mayo Clinic in Rochester, Minnesota, have transitioned to organize care around the patient and their specific clinical problem. Everyone working in a specific area is oriented toward creating the best results for each patient, as well as pursuing continuous quality improvement in the process. Furthermore, these institutions foster physician leadership. They look to promote physicians who are still actively involved in care delivery, so the administrative team does not get disconnected from the actual delivery of care.

Applying an EOC-based approach to common surgical problems, such as treating hernias, is fairly straightforward. However, it can just as easily be applied to other clinical situations. Hospital admissions for specific medical and psychiatric problems also lend themselves to an EOC-based approach. A patient develops a specific clinical problem. This problem requires an accurate diagnosis and a clear treatment plan. This treatment plan then needs to be carried out by a dedicated service line team in a coordinated manner.

Even chronic conditions lend themselves to a service line approach to treatment. By reframing a chronic condition—such as high blood pressure, diabetic management, or renal failure—as a time-based episode (for example, over three months, six months, or a year), chronic disease management of complex problems can be seen through the EOC lens.

Fortunately, there are a finite number of categories of medical problems (Table 5), allowing for the development of service lines that can manage most of the clinical conditions encountered within a healthcare system.

Table 5: Possible Team-Based Clinical Service Lines

Cardiac
Pulmonary
Abdominal
     Colon/Rectal
     Liver
     Abdominal wall/hernia
Vascular
Renal
Neurologic
Musculoskeletal
     Spinal
     Upper extremity
          Shoulder
          Elbow
          Hand
     Lower extremity
          Hip (including joint replacements)
          Knee (including joint replacements)
          Foot and ankle
Acute/Trauma
          General surgical trauma
          Neurosurgical trauma
          Musculoskeletal trauma
Hospitalist service line (acute in-hospital medical care)
Oncology service line
Mental Health / Psychiatric service line

Transforming the Canadian healthcare system also requires a fundamental structural reorganization with respect to how it manages patients with more complex and involved medical problems (surgeries, hospital admissions, complex chronic medical problems, etc.). The *second pathway* option being proposed integrates multidisciplinary teams, oriented around specific clinical problems and the associated EOC. These teams (service lines or programs) would work closely with the PCMHs. Various teams could be gradually added to the system until all clinical conditions were covered by at least one service line.

The structure of these teams would be akin to what the Shouldice Clinic has been doing for more than a half-century—organizing care delivery around specific types of clinical problems and the patients who have these problems. Teams would have the following elements:

1. *Multidisciplinary teams would be oriented around specific service lines.*
2. *Population-based healthcare goals would be established for each team.*
3. *Funding would occur via bundled payments for each EOC rendered.*
4. *Physicians and other team members would be hired by the service line*
5. *Teams would embrace and fully incorporate accepted business practices.*
6. *Teams would incorporate ongoing initiatives regarding quality and process improvement.*
7. *Individual team members would be held accountable for performance standards.*
8. *Accurate outcome measures would be collected to assess overall team performance.*
9. *Service lines would compete against each other.*

1. Multidisciplinary teams would be oriented around specific service lines.

All individuals required to run a specific service line (including physicians, nurses, therapists, administrators, and even housecleaners) would serve together on the same team. In addition to daily collaboration and informal, team-member communication, regular team meetings would be held. All team members (including physicians) would be required to attend, in person or virtually. These meetings would provide a venue for *all* team members to discuss team goals, outstanding issues, and the results of the care that has previously been delivered.

Teams would be large enough to allow for all aspects of care to be delivered within that particular service line, but small enough that everyone would be expected to be on a first-name basis with everyone else on the team. The roles and responsibility of all team members would be known. Therefore, when some action was required to improve overall clinical performance, it would be clear who could facilitate these changes. The team leader would be ultimately responsible for facilitating patient care. He or she would be clinically active and intimately involved with all aspects of the care delivery process.

While most team members would work full-time for one service line team or program, in some instances, individuals could work with multiple service line teams—or a service line team *and* a care facility (e.g., a hospital) team. For example, an orthopaedic surgeon might be contracted to be part of the "shoulder service line team" and also be affiliated with the "trauma or acute care" service line. Similarly, a housecleaner might be affiliated with a specific service line but also have a formal responsibility to a hospital team. In situations where an individual is affiliated with multiple teams, this affiliation should ideally be complementary and should never create a conflict in providing the necessary work performance for either team.

2. Population-based healthcare goals would be established for each team.

The type of clinical conditions—and the volume of patients with these conditions that each team would be expected to manage in a given year—will be established by population-based analyses. The governing body of each healthcare system should be able to calculate, with a high degree of accuracy, the specific clinical needs for this patient population each year. Each team will be given a clear mandate by the health system's governing body and be expected to accept the responsibility for serving the community that it is working in. Understanding the specific healthcare needs of that community, with respect to their clinical service line, allows each team to accurately predict what services they will need to provide.

Teams would often have a mandate to facilitate care over a wide geographical area –including ensuring adequate access to specialty care in rural populations. A *service line* team may be based in a central location, but it would be common to extend the *program* over a wide area by establishing satellite offices or mobile clinics. In addition, proactive care and community education would be part of the team's mandate. Ultimately, each service line team would exist to meet the healthcare needs of the population it serves.

3. Funding would occur via bundled payments for each EOC rendered.

Teams would generate revenue based, in large part, on set bundled payments for each EOC. It may be necessary to provide some upfront base payments to help establish each program. However, the number of successful EOCs they delivered would determine the total yearly funding that each service line team or program received.

Funding would also be tied to patient satisfaction scores, outcome metrics, and complication rates. Simply providing the service would not be enough to ensure funding. Services would need to meet certain standards. Furthermore, avoidable complications, such as post-operative infections that resulted in increased expenses to the system, would be charged to the programs.

This type of funding model would encourage excellence and efficiency. If a service line ran well, there would be ample funding to pay salaries (or offer contracted positions) to those affiliated with the service line—including providing productivity and performance bonuses to key healthcare workers.

4. Physicians and other team members would be hired by the service line.

Team members for each service line or program IPU would be hired by the IPU. This would include physicians who would either be salaried or contracted. Traditional fee-for-service compensation would be eliminated for those physicians working for the service line.

However, salaried physicians as well as IPU administrators would be eligible for regular bonuses based on objective measures of productivity, quality, and patient satisfaction. A baseline level of productivity, and performance standards would be clearly outlined in any job description for physicians and others employed by the service line. This approach to compensation is designed to allow the program to ensure it has adequate resources to carry out its clinical mandate for the governing body.

5. Teams would embrace and fully incorporate accepted business practices.

It would be expected that each service line team would take a very businesslike approach to meeting their care delivery needs. Commonly accepted business principles would be used to improve efficiency, increase team members' job satisfaction, and ultimately improve patient care.

A strong emphasis would be placed on decreasing practice variation. In a production or service process, decreased variation is known to correlate with higher quality. Among the strategies for decreasing variation would be the development of standardized clinical pathways. In addition, ongoing analysis of variations and their potential sources would be regularly reviewed.

6. Teams would incorporate ongoing initiatives regarding quality and process improvement.

Similar to the strategy proposed for PCMHs in the previous subsection, each service line team would have a quality improvement subgroup. This group would include the leader of the service line team and representatives of all team members. Strategies such as lean thinking, Six Sigma, total quality management (TQM), root cause analysis (RCA), and failure mode effects analysis (as outlined in Chapter 6) would be employed. Regular quality-improvement projects would be initiated.

Through the weekly meetings, as well as informal discussion among the team members, every member of the service line team would develop an understanding of quality and process improvement. A culture would be fostered, whereby every team member would be looking to improve the overall care and would not hesitate to bring suggestions forward to the larger group.

7. Individual team members would be held accountable for performance standards.

The multidisciplinary service line team would be expected to work in an integrated and coordinated manner. However, each individual would be held accountable for his or her job responsibilities. Individuals who are not fulfilling their specific roles would be reviewed. If a process issue was identified, it would be addressed by the administrative leaders. However, if the issue were one of inadequate job performance, then the employee would need to be remediated or terminated. Every team member would be held accountable for his or her job responsibilities.

8. Accurate outcome measures would be collected to assess overall team performance.

Independently-collected outcome metrics that delineate the results of the service line would be regularly obtained. These would include patient satisfaction scores, clinical results, complication rates, and per capita costs. This data would serve as the impetus for maintaining and improving the performance of the service line team. All members of the team would be regularly apprised of how patients were doing clinically, as well as the overall results of the outcome metrics that were obtained.

Just as a professional hockey team pays close attention to how they are doing in the standings, it would be expected that the service line team members would pay close attention to their outcome metrics. The accurate, objective nature of these outcome metrics would serve as concrete feedback to the group. For high-performing teams, it would also be expected that these outcome metrics would be a source of pride for all team members.

9. Service lines would compete against each other.

In most health systems, there would be more than one service line, and often, there would be many service lines devoted to the same clinical condition. Given that each of the service lines would be subject to identical, independent outcome metrics, it would be expected that comparisons between the service line teams would be the norm. Competition would be encouraged; however, this would also be combined with transparency. Solutions that work for one team would be shared with other service line teams.

In the event that one team performed at a substantially lower level than other teams, that service line would be placed on probation. If a team failed to improve to acceptable levels during the probationary period, that team would be disbanded. Probation would likely be applied to 10-15% of teams. While disbanding an existing service line team would be considered uncommon, it would be likely that between 2-5% of service line teams would suffer this fate.

It is essential that these punitive actions be implemented. Without the possibility of negative consequences, poorly performing teams would not have the adequate incentives to improve.

Facilities: Hospitals and other sites where healthcare is delivered

A professional hockey team needs first-class facilities—a place to practice and an arena to play their games in. Their fans need comfortable seats, high-quality concessions, good public transportation, and accessible parking. The home facility needs to be run by a team of coordinated employees—ticket collectors, ushers, concession workers, a security team, and a maintenance team to keep the building and the ice in top form. Similarly, a healthcare team needs high-quality facilities to carry out its work.

Professional hockey teams often lease their arenas. This gives them the opportunity to move when the facility no longer serves their needs. Hockey teams work closely with the facility's staff. However, those running the facility are usually a separate group of employees with their own management—set apart from the players, coaches, and trainers that work specifically for the hockey team.

Similarly, high-quality healthcare teams need to work closely with the facilities where they carry out their patient care—hospitals, clinics, and surgery centres. However, just as in professional hockey, it makes sense to keep the teams and the facilities separate. This gives healthcare teams the option of moving to other facilities if they are not receiving the service and performance they need to provide high-quality patient care.

These facilities represent the healthcare playing field. They are the fourth broad category of the *second pathway* healthcare system being proposed. Healthcare facilities need to be designed, staffed, and administered to provide high-quality, efficient service to the healthcare teams that are using their facilities. In many instances, the teams and the facilities will be intimately related, such as a medical ward on a hospital that is staffed by an inpatient medicine service line. In other instances, they will serve as regular hosts to a healthcare team, such as a shoulder program that operates at an outpatient surgery centre twice a week.

However, in each instance, the healthcare delivery team and the facilities should be separate. This creates competition. It gives the healthcare team the option of moving to a different facility if they're not satisfied with the performance they are receiving. Similarly, it gives the hospital or other facility being used, an opportunity to exclude an underperforming or financially inefficient healthcare team. Competition based on value is critical, in order to drive performance in a modern healthcare system.

For those running facilities, there are a series of basic principles that should guide their actions. These principles are:

1. *Facilities need to be customer-centred.*
2. *Competition should drive the performance of healthcare facilities.*
3. *Cleanliness is the canary in the coalmine.*
4. *Equipment and physical plants must be kept up-to-date.*
5. *Facilities require strong leadership and a skilled management team.*
6. *Facilities must be financially viable.*

1. Facilities need to be customer-centred.

The facility's customers are the various healthcare teams practicing at their premises—and by extension the patients these healthcare team are treating. As such, hospitals and other facilities must focus on the specific needs of their customers. This includes being acutely attuned to what those needs are, and it means being realistic about which needs they can meet and which they cannot.

2. Competition should drive the performance of healthcare facilities.

The proposed second pathway to healthcare reform is predicated on competition—even if the competition is internal (i.e., within the public system). Better performing facilities will garner more contracts by offering healthcare teams and programs the capacity to choose where their patients receive surgical care, hospital admission, or outpatient treatment. Poorer-performing facilities will be forced to reform or face extinction—or at a minimum, wholesale management change.

3. Cleanliness is the canary in the coalmine.[198]

Healthcare facilities must be clean. Since Lister describe the practical applications of the germ theory in the 1870s, it has been known that facilities where healthcare is delivered need to be kept meticulously clean. This is especially critically for hospitals providing surgical care and treating patients who are acutely ill. Ensuring cleanliness is not always easy. Illness can be a messy business; bacteria and viruses can be easily transmitted between patients via healthcare providers and cleaning staff that are not hyper vigilant.

However, effective strategies for keeping a healthcare facility clean are well known. Ensuring these strategies are fully implemented is essential for those running a healthcare facility. How a hospital or other facility ensures cleanliness is a microcosm for other performance issues. A hospital that keeps its facility clean at all times, has an informed staff, and maintains a proactive approach to ensure safety will almost

---

[198] The expression "the canary in the coalmine" is in reference to an early sign of an impending problem. For years coalminers would take canaries down into the mines with them while they worked. As long as the canaries were alive and chirping the miners knew they were safe from poisonous gases such as carbon monoxide. However, if the birds became unresponsive the minors knew they needed to exit the mines immediately.

invariably perform well in other areas. Those facilities that cannot maintain basic standards of cleanliness will likely struggle in other aspects of the performance of facility care delivery.

4. Equipment and physical plants must be kept up-to-date.

Providing the physical facilities, the equipment, and the support personnel is the primary mandate for healthcare facilities. Those running these facilities must realize this responsibility. Equipment, which can be as diverse as operating room instruments, ventilators for the ICU, and hospital beds, must all be functioning. Staff must know where this equipment is located—and how it works.

Additionally, the physical facility must be well maintained. Elevators need to be working, the air filtration system should be regularly monitored, and the building itself should be maintained. To do this requires recognition that equipment and physical structures break down over time. It may not be possible to predict when a particular piece of equipment will fail, or when a section of the facility will need to be renovated; but collectively, it is possible to know that these expenses will occur on a regular basis and therefore need to be budgeted for.

5. Facilities require strong leadership and a skilled management team.

Successful operation of facilities, like healthcare teams, requires clear goals, the hiring of personnel that work in a coordinated and effective manner, a customer-focused approach, and the collection of accurate, prospective performance data (including income and expenses). To do this requires clear leadership and a strong management team. It also demands that facility leaders think and act proactively to meet the needs of future customers, and to gain new business opportunities.

The ultimate success of a healthcare facility, such as a hospital, is dependent on having the right leaders. These leaders need to be held accountable for the performance of the facility. This means providing excellent compensation to those leadership teams that are successful and bringing in new leadership teams for those that are not. A more businesslike approach, including possibly hiring successful business executives to lead some of these facilities, is likely to be required.

6. Facilities must be financially viable.

Healthcare facilities must be run as businesses with strong leadership and management. Healthcare teams and the patients they serve will be expecting various facilities to compete against each other, based on performance and cost. Similarly, facilities should only take on contracts from programs that make sense to them financially. There are many costs related to the physical plant, associated equipment, and personnel, which are required to successfully run a healthcare facility. These costs need to be accurately assessed and built into the larger management plan for the facility.

Summary: Chapter 9

This chapter has explored potential solutions for reforming the Canadian healthcare system. Consider a last-place, professional hockey team. Going from last place to winning the Stanley Cup is not an easy road. However, one can imagine multiple decisions over many years that create steady, incremental improvement. A few of the many areas that would need to be emphasized are strong draft choices, a commitment to an effective style of play, fostering team chemistry, and consistently placing the values of team excellence over individual goals.

This rise to excellence would be a challenge. Every other team in the league is attempting to do the same thing. However, it is possible. There is an existing structure within the NHL that makes this feasible. There is an established hierarchy of priorities. The NHL's head office does what they believe to be in the best interest of the league as a whole, trumping the individual interests of various teams. In turn, team goals trump the respective interests of the individual players.

This hierarchy was not always present in professional hockey. The early days of professional hockey in Canada saw individuals moving from team to team, as well as teams themselves dominating the league office. However, since the consolidation of the NHL in the 1930s, this hierarchy (League>Teams>Individuals) has predominated.

In the Canadian healthcare system, there is no such hierarchy. If anything, the predominant *hierarchy* is essentially reversed. Doctors, the main players of the healthcare system, are de facto individual businesspeople, and as such, they can be expected to make the decisions that make the most sense for them individually. The teams they work with are really only loosely-affiliated groups—organized around siloed departments, rather than integrated service lines or programs. Even where specific programs exist, physicians are usually still able to act with autonomy. The governing bodies of each healthcare system, whether they be provincial health ministries or regional health authorities, rarely function with central authority—at least not akin to the way the NHL head office does.

Despite this dysfunctionally inverted hierarchy of authority, there is room for meaningful, evolutionary change –and in isolated cases some of these changes are occurring. A concerted effort—to incorporate as many of the principles of modern healthcare that are outlined in Chapter 8 as possible—will lead to noticeable improvements in the existing healthcare system. Furthermore, the present manifestation of the Canadian healthcare system will not disappear quickly, so emphasis should be given to the types of evolutionary changes suggested.

However, steady incremental change within the Canadian healthcare system will never alter the fact that the foundation of the system is fundamentally flawed. One means of addressing this reality has been outlined in this chapter—a *second pathway* built new from the foundation up—based on the principles of 21st century healthcare delivery. This new system would in many ways mirror the modern NHL: strong central leadership from the head office, as well as teams that are oriented toward outcomes and work as a unit—where team goals supersede those of individual players.

This second system would have four elements. The primary element would be a governing body akin to the role of the NHL head office. This organization would set goals based on the population's healthcare needs. There would be two variations of healthcare *teams*. One set of teams would focus on delivering high-quality primary care, representing

~90% of the patient care provided by the healthcare system. A second set of teams would be organized to address more complex, specific clinical problems—service line or program teams. The final element would be facilities: hospitals, outpatient clinics, surgery centers, and any other place where healthcare services are delivered. These facilities would be administered and managed in a highly-organized manner—similar to how a hockey arena is run for each professional team.

This new system would be true to the principles of 21st century medicine. It would focus on delivering high-value healthcare by promoting internal competition. This *second pathway* public healthcare system would need to be run in a manner that ensures it remained at arm's length from government interference (ex. as a Crown corporation). It could start relatively small—perhaps 5% of the provincial healthcare budget. However, as it would be oriented toward quality and performance as determined by the system's customers (patients and taxpayers), it would steadily gain popularity and, by extension, market share.

Administered effectively and remaining true to its founding principles, it would overtake and surpass the existing system in time, leading to the eventual extinction of what we now know as the present-day Canadian healthcare system. Canadians would be left with a modern public healthcare system that delivers the care they need at a fair price. It would fully embody the ideals of Canadian healthcare: universal access and full government funding. In addition, it would add a third element that is presently missing: high-value healthcare.

<u>Summary Points: Chapter 9</u>

There are two types of system change: *evolutionary change* and *disruptive change*. Evolutionary change occurs when a system gradually and steadily improves in an incremental fashion. Disruptive change is characterized by the introduction of a completely new paradigm.

The existing Canadian healthcare system will benefit from both kinds of change. Incremental improvements should be promoted in a coordinated manner in an attempt to optimize the traditional healthcare system. However, the existing system is based on a model of funding and organizing care that generates multiple roadblocks to high-quality, high-value healthcare delivery.

The flawed design of the existing Canadian healthcare system creates a powerful argument for disruptive change. To facilitate this type of change, this chapter advocates for the creation of an entirely new second, parallel public healthcare system built from the ground up based on the principles of modern medicine that have been previously outlined. As quality and efficiency gains from an appropriately designed and implemented second system are realized, it would steadily supplant the existing system over time.

CONCLUSION

Canadians are passionately supportive of their healthcare system. The ideals of the system, which include universal access, comprehensive care, and public funding, have become a microcosm of Canadian values. However, Canadians are now seeing mounting evidence that increasingly demonstrates what those who objectively study the system have known for years—there is a chasm between these ideals and the reality of the system. Healthcare in Canada is prohibitively expensive, but despite this, it struggles to consistently deliver even mediocre care.

Notwithstanding their passionate feelings, most Canadians spend little time thinking about healthcare. Collectively, they spend more time talking about and analyzing the exploits of their favorite NHL hockey team. This is unfortunate. The truth is that when Canadians are injured or become seriously ill, they will need to rely on this fragmented, often uncoordinated system for the care they receive.

The central thesis of this book is that the Canadian healthcare system needs fundamental reform to ensure that patients receive consistently high-value care and that the system has long-term sustainability. To achieve this reform requires a major, structural reorganization of the system. The present system is not a system at all. Rather, it is a means of funding hospital care and physician services. The predominant nature of this funding model (bulk funding of hospitals and fee-for-service funding of physicians) is based on the quirks of history, rather than practical realities. Why not build a truly integrated system—the way it should have been built in the first place?

A central premise of this book has been that there are well-established principles of organizing and delivering high-value 21st century medical care, and these principles should be invoked in any health system reform. The NHL provides an analogy for how healthcare delivery should be organized. They have a governing body that oversees the various teams and sets the agenda for the league—with a primary agenda of improving the overall wellbeing of the league itself. Likewise, successful health systems need a strong governing body to set clear goals and ensure the health system's agenda is carried out. In order to achieve success, NHL teams require a highly-coordinated effort among the players with outstanding coaching and management. Players know their roles, and recognize that their individual goals are subservient to the larger goals of the team.

Similarly, high-quality 21st century healthcare is now a team event. The goals of the healthcare team must trump the individual goals of the various healthcare players (doctors, nurses, administrators, etc.). Many of these principles for team success are self-evident: have clear goals, work as a team, hold individuals accountable, and continuously make improvements based on outcomes. These are principles that every successful professional hockey team uses to optimize their success.

Unfortunately, consistently invoking these team-oriented principles is difficult or impossible in the existing healthcare system. The fee-for-service funding model promotes individual-oriented physician behavior, while yearly bulk funding of hospitals stifles creativity. The existing system works well for many healthcare players, as flawed as it might be for patients and taxpayers. Physicians, administrators, and other healthcare workers have often carved out well-compensated niches within the system, which they protect ferociously. A profound change to the existing system is not likely to be successful if it competes directly with these powerful groups.

However, fundamental reform of the Canadian healthcare system is possible. To institute this type of disruptive healthcare innovation requires that a second public healthcare system be developed—a system run as a Crown corporation at arm's length from direct government interference, but that still includes full government oversight. This second system must be predicated on a commitment to adhere to established principles for providing excellent, coordinated, team-based healthcare delivery. And it demands an organizational structure that puts patients and taxpayers first.

There are a variety of potential manifestations of such a system. In general, a focus on principles and structure is required, rather than a dogmatic approach to a predetermined structure. By correctly building a new healthcare system from the foundation up, high-quality healthcare could be achieved at a fraction of the present cost. Over time as this second system grows, it would supplant the existing system, ultimately leaving Canada with the first-rate healthcare system it deserves.

The impetus for these sorts of fundamental changes will not come from within the existing healthcare system, nor are they likely to arise de novo from the provincial or federal governments. They will only come about when an informed and passionate population pushes their leaders to institute such changes. Canadians believe in the ideals of their healthcare system; now they need to push to transform these ideals into reality. Like passionate and knowledgeable hockey fans, they need to prod the overseers of their healthcare system to do better.

This book serves to provide Canadians who cherish the ideals of a high-functioning, publicly-funded healthcare system with a roadmap for achieving the system Canada deserves.

ACKNOWLEDGMENTS

Writing a book is a journey —a prolonged adventure that inevitably requires help and support to complete. I am tremendously grateful to the countless patients and healthcare providers who have been willing to talk to me openly and honestly about their views on the Canadian healthcare system. I have learned much from their experiences and various perspectives.

Numerous friends, colleagues, and experts gave freely of their time, energy, and support. They made this adventure possible —and enjoyable. My friend Professor Naoko Ellis encouraged me to start this project and was a steady source of support throughout. I am grateful for her patience and clear thinking. Dr. Selena Lawrie graciously gave her time and knowledge serving as a content editor and an invaluable sounding board on multiple occasions —a process that not only improved the final product, but also made the experience fun. Professor Jason Sutherland was kind enough to review this work. His expertise led to multiple insightful comments that were of tremendous help in shaping the final version of the book. Comments and suggestions from my colleague Dr. Joseph Bernstein were invaluable. Professor Lisa Surridge provided expert and timely feedback. I was also fortunate to have ongoing support and wonderful input from my friend and academic collaborator Professor Anita Ho. Her analysis and deft editing touch was of great benefit.

In editing and revising this book I had expert help. Tom Johnson provided excellent copyediting. His efficiency and expertise was greatly appreciated. I am particularly grateful to my outstanding editor Michelle Josette. Her creativity, attention to detail, and expertise were invaluable in producing the final version of this book.

My thanks also go out to Professor Dan Pratt who has been a long-time friend and adviser. He taught me the importance observing and understanding multiple perspectives, an essential quality when confronting the complexities of our healthcare system. I benefited from the wisdom and experience of the late Dr. Cy Frank. He was a mentor to me —and to a generation of Canadian orthopaedic surgeons. He is greatly missed, but his ideas and vision live on. I would also like to thank my friends Paul Roache, Russell Long, Kimberly Ota, and Savita Chand whose support and encouragement was greatly appreciated during the many months I spent researching and writing this book. Finally, I owe a debt of gratitude to my father Baden Pinney not only for his support, but also for his excellent editing suggestions and constructive criticism.

INDEX

C

Canada Health Act 20, 56, 105,
    107, 108, 110, 111, 113, 118
  accessibility 109, 110
  comprehensiveness 109
  portability 107, 109
  public administration 107, 109
  universality 109
Canada Health Transfer (CHT) 10
Canadian Broadcasting Corporation
    (CBC) 238
Canadian healthcare system xiv–xx,
    4–5, 7–8, 10, 12–14, 19–21,
    32, 39–46, 53–54, 57–58, 83,
    86, 92, 95–116, 122, 130, 134,
    143, 145, 152–153, 160, 161,
    165–166, 171, 175–176, 182,
    194–195, 195, 200, 204–205,
    208, 213, 218–219, 226–233,
    262–264
  1800s 66, 67, 69, 71, 72, 73, 92, 93,
    94, 118, 195
  1950s and 1960s 79, 81
  Canada Health Act to the Romanow
    Report (1985-2002) 110
  curtain 10, 12, 16, 226
  Depression and World War II 96
  dysfunctional system xv, 12
  early 1900s 63, 89, 95
  fragmented system 59
  history xiv, xvi, 3, 16, 57, 62, 63, 65,
    66, 68, 71, 76, 77, 89, 92, 93, 96,
    97, 102, 104, 117, 118, 152, 171,
    181, 207, 267
  idealized view xvii, 11, 39, 111
  lack of competition 43, 56, 59, 61
  Medicare to the Canada Health Act
    (1968-1984) 105
  perverse incentive 59
  private xix, xx, 14, 20, 39, 56, 57, 95,
    103, 113, 114, 117, 159, 163,
    229, 230
  provincial jurisdiction 117, 118

  reforming xvii, xix, 134, 191, 213,
    218, 226, 234, 262
  Romanow Report (2002-Present)
    114
  sanitation 95, 117, 118
  second system 263, 267, 268, 269
Canadian Hockey Association
    (CHA) 89
Canadian Institute for Health
    Information (CIHI) 185,
    231
Canadian Medical Association
    (CMA) 97, 102
  Economic Committee 97
Canadian National Council for
    Combating Venereal Diseases
    96
canary in the coalmine 259, 260
Carnegie Foundation 67
cataract surgery 218
central line infections 131
change xvi, 9, 11, 12, 14, 23, 31,
    44–45, 48, 50–51, 85–86,
    100, 102, 115, 126, 133, 140,
    188, 194–196, 198, 213–216,
    226–227, 229, 232–233, 237,
    246–247, 254, 260
  disruptive xvii, 23, 117, 195, 196,
    216, 225, 226, 227, 232, 237,
    250, 265, 268
  evolutionary 170, 195, 198, 226, 227,
    263, 265
Checklist Manifesto, The 85
Checklist(s)
  surgical x, xiii, xv, 4, 5, 7, 8, 9, 12, 18,
    23, 24, 28, 30, 43, 44, 45, 46, 47,
    50, 51, 55, 56, 57, 60, 73, 74, 77,
    79, 80, 81, 83, 95, 99, 100, 113,
    118, 120, 127, 134, 135, 136,
    139, 160, 161, 163, 164, 165,
    169, 172, 174, 175, 185, 187,
    188, 193, 197, 251, 252, 260
Chrétien, Prime Minister Jean 114

New Democratic Party 102
New England Journal of Medicine 133
nitrous oxide 72
Nobel Prize 78, 99
North American Surgical Quality Improvement Program (NSQIP) 50
nurses xv, xvii, 7, 14, 15, 27, 28, 29, 32, 38, 42, 43, 44, 45, 48, 49, 50, 61, 84, 101, 120, 133, 145, 153, 161, 162, 163, 165, 183, 187, 189, 204, 208, 210, 212, 215, 228, 238, 240, 245, 253, 268
nursing homes 20, 101

O

obstetrics 66, 68, 76
one problem per visit 52
Ontario Professional Hockey League (OPHL) 89
operating room (OR) 15
  OR nurses 15, 44
orphan patients 30
orthopaedic surgeon xv, 52, 53, 56, 57, 58, 59, 154, 159, 162, 189, 197, 254
  graduates 57, 66, 113
  worst 56, 57, 59
Osler, Sir William 65
Ostry, Alec 100, 101
outcome metrics 42, 49, 50, 51, 58, 61, 116, 142, 169, 184, 185, 186, 208, 209, 217, 227, 228, 230, 231, 232, 234, 235, 239, 240, 248, 249, 255, 257, 258
outputs 14, 16, 32, 33, 37, 139, 147, 153, 162, 170, 179, 184, 186, 187, 218, 223, 234
  definition 186, 188, 196, 201, 217

pay for 25, 26, 32, 33, 37, 60, 61, 97, 104, 147, 153, 170, 179, 186, 223
Owners 14, 56, 63, 89, 91, 116, 117, 171, 184, 213

P

Pacific Coast Hockey League 90
parallel public system xvii, 233
pasteurization 73
Pasteur, Louis 73
pathologist 4, 76
pathology 3, 4, 66, 68, 79
patient and family centred care (PFCC) 136
patient care 7, 15, 28, 29, 42, 46, 58, 61, 66, 67, 101, 152, 153, 167, 187, 191, 196, 202, 203, 204, 224, 240, 251, 254, 256, 259, 264
  mediocre xiv, 9, 10, 35, 37, 42, 43, 44, 58, 60, 61, 116, 238, 267
  siloed xiv, 9, 13, 15, 32, 42, 44, 58, 61, 141, 167, 263
  team-based xvi, 13, 14, 42, 45, 54, 60, 61, 69, 86, 88, 101, 117, 137, 143, 158, 160, 161, 163, 167, 172, 178, 182, 183, 200, 201, 205, 211, 212, 215, 232, 234, 236, 240, 242, 244, 245, 246, 251, 252, 268
patient-centred x, 25, 40, 48, 125, 126, 140, 141, 146, 152, 158, 169, 179, 182, 196, 202, 203, 219, 220, 223, 224, 235, 236, 239, 242, 248
patient-centred medical homes (PCMH) 235, 236, 242
  leadership xv, 48, 60, 93, 101, 102, 103, 106, 148, 162, 171, 176, 178, 181, 202, 206, 207, 215, 217, 218, 222, 224, 232, 236, 237, 238, 242, 246, 250, 251, 259, 261, 262, 263

system change xv, 237, 265
system within a system xvii

T

taxpayers xiv, xvii, xix, 5, 8, 14, 19,
    32, 39, 61, 129, 146, 171, 179,
    180, 181, 200, 214, 222, 223,
    264, 268, 269
teams xvi–xviii, 13, 25, 59–60,
    116–117, 141–148, 152,
    157–164, 167–171, 176–178,
    182–184, 193, 198, 200–217,
    221–222, 227, 232, 234–236,
    239, 240–246, 250–264
  physician-led 13, 242
telemedicine 244, 245, 247
tests 55, 83, 121, 139, 155, 186, 191,
    194
  CT scan 52, 92
  MRI x, 4, 38, 154, 158, 159, 181
  x-rays 3, 4, 6, 37, 38, 121, 186, 191
too big to fail 179, 193, 194, 224,
    227, 229, 235
transparency xx, 7, 19, 23, 26, 27, 32,
    34, 35, 51, 159, 160, 180, 198,
    199, 222, 224, 228, 258
triple aim 127, 129, 130, 138, 144,
    247
True North Sports and
    Entertainment (TNSE) 213
twilight zone 45, 46, 47, 48, 49, 58

U

United States xiv, xv, xix, 11, 27, 39,
    40, 50, 57, 67, 68, 71, 75, 83,
    84, 85, 113, 119, 122, 123,
    125, 177
  healthcare system xix, 39–41, 82–84,
    125

University of British Columbia xiv,
    23
University of Pennsylvania 65
urinary tract infections (UTIs) 49
urologist 52, 53
user fees xx, 100, 106, 107

V

value xvi, xx, 13, 21, 26, 33, 39, 61,
    114, 116, 137, 139, 140, 143,
    144, 145, 146, 147, 148, 159,
    176, 180, 183, 187, 190, 200,
    202, 203, 205, 210, 212, 215,
    216, 218, 223, 224, 230, 235,
    239, 246, 259, 264, 265, 267
  high value 13, 21, 33
value agenda 140, 147
variations xix, 23, 83, 144, 157, 183,
    192, 211, 219, 256, 263
  decreasing variation 83, 135, 136,
    183, 192, 193, 256
  in care 23, 35, 54, 55, 83, 141, 144,
    181, 230, 235, 251
  utilization 23, 29, 231

W

Wait time 55, 56, 159, 160, 174,
    175, 182
Watanabe, Dr. Masaki 81
Wells, Horace 72
Who Operates When (WOW II)
    46
work arounds 14, 16
wrong-sided surgery 8, 9

X

x-rays 3, 4, 6, 37, 38, 121, 186, 191